THE CASINO SHIFT

THE CASINO SHIFT

STORIES FROM AN ER ON THE EDGE

BRIAN GOLDMAN, MD

Collins

The Casino Shift

Published by Collins, an imprint of HarperCollins Publishers Ltd

FIRST EDITION

This book describes or quotes actual patients or healthcare colleagues only with permission. Otherwise, the author's stories of patients and first-name-only colleagues are composites drawn from many the author has encountered in his long career in emergency medicine. The same is true of stories from his quoted colleagues.

This book does not provide medical advice.

HarperCollins Publishers Ltd
Bay Adelaide Centre, East Tower
22 Adelaide Street West, 41st Floor
Toronto, Ontario, Canada
M5H 4E3

www.harpercollins.ca

HarperCollins Publishers
Macken House, 39/40 Mayor Street Upper
Dublin 1, D01 C9W8, Ireland
https://www.harpercollins.com

Library and Archives Canada Cataloguing in Publication

Title: The casino shift : stories from an ER on the edge / Brian Goldman, MD.
Names: Goldman, Brian, author
Identifiers: Canadiana (print) 20250316390 | Canadiana (ebook) 20250316404 | ISBN 9781443473583 (hardcover) | ISBN 9781443473590 (EPUB)
Subjects: LCSH: Goldman, Brian—Anecdotes. | LCSH: Hospitals—Emergency services—Canada—Anecdotes. | LCSH: Emergency medicine—Canada—Anecdotes. | LCSH: Emergency physicians—Canada—Anecdotes. | LCSH: Emergency medical personnel—Canada—Anecdotes. | LCSH: Emergency medicine—Popular works. | LCGFT: Anecdotes.
Classification: LCC RA975.5.E5 G63 2026 | DDC 362.180971—dc23

Printed and bound in the United States of America

26 27 28 29 30 LBC 6 5 4 3 2

To the smart, resourceful, kind and dedicated
ER colleagues young and young at heart
that I've worked with over my career.

Contents

INTRODUCTION

6:25 p.m.

"Dr. Goldman, it's the emergency department calling," says an ER ward clerk named Vivica.

At the dinner table, my family sees me flinch.

"Sorry to bother you, but the department is backing up," says Vivica. "We're hoping you can come in early."

There are times I want to let these calls go to voicemail, but our group of ER physicians long ago agreed to pitch in and arrive as early as two hours before the start of a scheduled shift when we're needed.

"It's no bother at all," I reply. "On my way."

The "no bother" bit is a fib. I don't like being called in early because it raises my stress level a tad prematurely. I don't get the time I need to transition from Sunday dinner with my wife, kids and mother-in-law to the high-stress environment of a downtown big-city ER.

The twenty-minute drive to the hospital gives me time to steady my nerves. As a chronic worrywart who has trouble sleeping, I try to stop myself from imagining the scene that awaits me. My usual fears include working too slowly to tackle the volume of patients waiting to be seen and missing the signs of a life-threatening condition.

When I arrive, I walk through the revolving door at the back entrance to the hospital and enter the lobby. To my right, close to the front entrance, sits the emergency room, separated from the lobby by a wall. But I head in the other direction, down to the ER physicians' offices, to change into blue scrubs. I never pass through the ER on my way to work because I don't want to see what awaits me until I'm ready to dive in.

The Casino Shift is the sequel to my first book, *The Night Shift: Real Life in the Heart of the ER*, which was published in 2010. In *The Night Shift*, I described the patients I saw over the course of one night, from ten until nine the next morning. The challenges faced by doctors who work nights are well known. Fatigue occurs after you've been up for sixteen hours or more. Working even one night, which means not sleeping when your body's clock says you're supposed to, puts you at odds with human circadian rhythms that have been honed by thousands of years of evolution. I've worked night shifts for four decades and found it stimulating for a lot of reasons but also difficult because of its physical and mental impacts.

Casino shifts are one tactic ERs are using to address those impacts. Not surprisingly, given the name, the idea was borrowed from casino employees, who typically work a six-hour shift, from 10:00 p.m. until 4:00 a.m. or from 4:00 a.m. until 10:00 a.m. The theory is that having two doctors split the twelve to fourteen hours of the night shift is better than having one work all night because it allows both MDs to sleep at least part of the night in their own beds when their bodies are telling them it's time to sleep.

In 2002, the first casino shifts in Canada were scheduled in the ER at the Queen Elizabeth II Health Sciences Centre in Halifax, Nova Scotia. This pilot project was overseen by Dr. Pat Croskerry, an ER physician and patient safety expert, and it found that the fifteen doctors involved said they slept more hours and had reduced sleep debt while enjoying better work performance and reduced cognitive impairment. The doctors also said the casino shift made them rethink quitting the ER, which many had been contemplating.

In the ER at my downtown Toronto hospital, where we see as many as two hundred patients a day, the casino shift begins at 9:00 p.m. and its end time is flexible. We still have a night shift doctor who starts at 11:00 p.m. and stops seeing incoming patients at 6:00 a.m., when the day physician starts work. Unlike the ER at the QEII Health Sciences Centre, we don't have a doctor arriving at 4:00 a.m.

Casino shifts are just one of many things that have changed in the ER since I wrote *The Night Shift*. The fifteen years since my first book was published have seen incredible leaps in technology. I now have a handheld ultrasound device that I carry in a fanny pack and can connect to my personal smartphone. It allows me to diagnose everything from heart failure to broken bones to shards of glass embedded in a patient's foot. In *The Night Shift*, I wrote at length about the challenge of learning how to insert an endotracheal, or breathing, tube into a patient's windpipe. Today, a tiny camera attached to the tube lets me see on a viewscreen exactly where I'm going. CT scans are now as plentiful as X-rays, and MRIs, once hard to get, are usually available within a day or two. With just a few keystrokes, I can access a patient's X-rays, blood work, diagnostic imaging reports and hospital discharge summaries in seconds.

The growth in know-how of ER physicians is also astonishing. I have colleagues who can read abdominal CT scans nearly on par with radiologists. We treat some gynecological conditions more often than gynecologists do. We assess and treat patients with emerging diseases like Ebola and dengue fever. (Although I've never seen a patient with Ebola, I've seen several with dengue.) We must be prepared to see, diagnose and treat any condition. We've also become experts in keeping critically ill patients alive.

There are more of us on duty at a time. I think most people would be surprised to hear this, because the conventional wisdom is that there's a doctor shortage. That's a recent issue I'll get into later, but when I started doing emergency medicine in the 1980s, I was the only doctor in the ER. Now, at peak times of the day, as many as four doctors are on shift. And it's not just ER physicians. We've also steadily increased the number of nurses on duty, and we've added nurse practitioners and physician assistants into the mix. We are also leveraging the knowledge and skills of physiotherapists, occupational therapists, speech and language pathologists, social workers, peer counsellors and pharmacists. We have embraced teamwork as never before.

But it's not all good news. The greying of our patient population is relentless. People come to the ER with eight or nine separate issues, and their problems are exponentially more complex than they were when I wrote *The Night Shift*. The ones with cancer may have had many operations and rounds of chemo and radiation. Many others take ten to twenty prescription medications. It takes a lot of extra time to assess and treat patients like these. I spend ten minutes or more at a computer terminal boning up on a patient's diagnostic and treatment history before I can even introduce myself.

Often, these patients require hospital admission. That would be manageable if the healthcare system had enough beds. But it doesn't. On that score, Canada ranks well below other industrialized nations. Sweden, Denmark and the Netherlands have fewer beds per capita, but they make up for the shortfall with innovative home care programs that Canada lacks.

A lot of beds are filled by patients with mental health conditions. Canada has a spotty record when it comes to community supports for people like this and ranks low against other nations in the number of psychiatrists and psychologists, as well as the number of psychiatric beds.

Increasingly, patients with mental health diagnoses come to the ER because they have no other place to go. That's true as well for the exploding number of people who live in precarious housing and those who have opioid use disorder and other addictions.

To these issues, you can add a new and growing problem that threatens to destabilize ERs across the country: Family doctors are quitting their practices like never before. Many are retiring, but younger ones, fed up with the relatively low pay (compared with specialists) and an ever-increasing burden of accountability paperwork, are walking away from family medicine. OurCare is a Toronto-based research group focused on problems in the healthcare system. A national survey it conducted in 2022, led by Dr. Tara Kiran at Unity Health Toronto, found that an estimated 6.5 million Canadians do not have a family physician or nurse practitioner they see regularly. That's up from 4.5 million in just three years. Not only that, but 60 per cent of those who do have primary care can't get a timely appointment. No primary care means much more than no treatment for minor ailments such as urinary tract infections. It means chronic ailments such as type 2 diabetes and high blood pressure go unmanaged for years or even decades, leading to preventable complications such as heart attacks, strokes and chronic kidney disease. In many provinces, it means no cancer screening.

Sooner or later, all of these "unattached" patients, as they are called, need healthcare. And when they do, they have two choices: They can go to walk-in clinics that fill their daily appointment slots within an hour of opening their doors, or they can go to the ER. Emergency departments have become the healthcare nexus point where patients who have no other place to go meet a system that has no place to put them. Increasingly, that puts ERs in the unenviable position of having the responsibility to take on all comers and little power to address chronic shortages in the system.

"I cannot add more long-term care beds," says Dr. Carolyn Snider, an ER physician and former chief of emergency medicine at St. Michael's Hospital in Toronto. "I cannot seem to change hospital flow on my own. Nobody allows us to say, 'No, shut the door,' but every other service is allowed to shut the door in Ontario. And that is an incredibly demoralizing environment to be in as an emergency physician, but especially as a leader."

When I was asked if I wanted to write a sequel to *The Night Shift*, I saw an incredible opportunity to give my take on emergency medicine as I inch closer to the end of my forty-plus years in the ER. Compared with the guy who wrote that first book, I'm much older and not nearly as fast as I once was. But what I bring to my work in the ER, to my time as host of *White Coat, Black Art* on CBC Radio One and to this book are wisdom, experience and a deep understanding of what makes ER people tick. What's more, I believe we're now at a critical inflection point: Either we define and fix what ails the ER and the system that surrounds it, or we turn out the lights and head towards an uncertain future that might well feature private for-profit healthcare.

This book is not a woeful tale of frustrated and burnt-out colleagues who can't wait to quit. Oh, I'll share with you the things in their daily work that fill them with thoughts of despair. But I will also share with you the passion they have for being there in your hour of greatest need. I'll bring you inspiring stories about diagnoses made, puzzles solved and lives saved.

The Casino Shift is an hour-by-hour account of what the ER is like in these turbulent times. But it's not a book about one shift at one hospital. Nor is the focus only on what ails the people we see in the ER. Rather, it's about what's happening in ERs big and small, urban and rural, close to the meccas of modern medicine and as remote as you can possibly imagine—and what these situations can tell us about the challenges facing the entire healthcare system in this country.

The patients you're about to meet are mostly composites of people I have seen and treated; the same is true for many of the doctors, nurses and other frontline providers portrayed here. The only actual patients and colleagues who appear have agreed to be included.

Buckle up. It's going to be a bumpy ride.

CHAPTER ONE

MOLLY

7:01 p.m.

There's chaos in the waiting room.

A glance at FirstNet, the app we use to track patients, shows that forty-three people have been triaged by nurses and are waiting to be seen. Nine have minor issues such as ankle sprains and sore eyes. Eight have intermediate problems such as abdominal pain and first-trimester bleeding. The other twenty-six have illnesses and injuries deemed major and in need of a full workup and a stretcher. It's far too many patients for my colleague Tawny to see. She started her shift at 6:00 p.m. That's why I've been called in early.

The start time for my casino shift was supposed to be 9:00 p.m. My job is to ride shotgun with the night doctor, who starts at eleven and is on the clock till the day physician arrives at six. I have no set quitting time. If it's quiet, I might be able to leave at around 2:00 a.m. That of course assumes things will stay that way. If it's busy, I'll stay as long as needed to see as many patients as possible and move them through the system. I can't predict which scenario I'll face on any given shift. It turns our casino shift into a game of chance.

"There were eighteen majors when I arrived," says Tawny as I enter the triage area. "I've seen nine and they just keep coming. I'm sorry I wasn't able to keep up."

"This isn't your fault," I tell her. As much as I'm ambivalent about being called in early, the last thing I want is to be the kind of ER doctor who makes a colleague feel inadequate for summoning the cavalry.

The triage area is one of the newest additions to the ER. It's a long, rectangular room. On my right, there's a bank of workstations for attending and trainee doctors, nurse practitioners and physician assistants, as well as one exclusively for the team leader, the nurse in charge. Tonight, that nurse is Cynthia. On my left, there's a plexiglass wall with five triage workstations to assess new patients. The plexiglass lets the nurses observe the waiting room at all times.

Two of the workstations are unstaffed.

"How many nurses are we short?" I ask Cynthia.

"Two," she replies. She's doing her team-leading duties while covering for the missing nurse at Triage 3.

Cynthia and I have worked together for more than ten years. She's old enough to be very experienced but young enough to still be young. If she thinks I'm past my prime, she doesn't show it. I like her for that. She's unflappable except when it comes to patients who are both emotional and noisy.

"Fire!" screams a dishevelled woman named Molly from atop a stretcher across the hall from the triage area. "Put out the fire!"

Molly is the type of patient we once called a "frequent flyer." The nickname has been abandoned because it's seen as pejorative and may encourage frontline workers to take these patients' very real emotional and clinical problems less seriously. Molly has chronic schizophrenia and a fixed delusion that someone has placed a tracking device in her belly. Despite this, she hasn't been admitted to a psychiatric hospital in years because she doesn't possess any of the red flags that would make doctors think she's a danger to herself or others. For instance, she doesn't hear voices compelling her to attack bystanders or jump from a bridge. She's homeless in large part because she's been kicked out of every shelter in downtown Toronto. She frequents ERs like ours when it's cold outside, as it is tonight.

"Somebody put out the fire!" she screams again.

When I first entered the triage area, I couldn't hear Molly's voice. Now it's all I can hear. And at this moment, her screeching voice is more than Cynthia can take.

"This is her third visit in three days," she says. "I know she's not first to be seen, but do you mind sorting her out now?"

"No problem," I say. I grab the chart and step through the plexiglass door and into the waiting room.

My anxiety about not being able to handle the crush of patients immediately begins to rise. Eight patients are waiting to register, and another five are waiting to be triaged. That's in addition to the dozens waiting to see me or one of my colleagues. It's more patients than we have beds, so for the time being, the waiting area will be my examining room.

The waiting area has the usual rows of chairs for people who can sit. Surrounding that are rooms for paramedics bearing patients on stretchers. They're always full. Molly is one of several patients on stretchers down a long hallway that connects to the waiting area and serves as a temporary holding space for additional paramedic stretchers. It all feels like a fishbowl. Every major patient waiting to be seen is outside the ER and crammed into the waiting area, people with pneumonia, chest pain, abdominal pain, bowel blockages and dizziness. Any one of them could be seriously ill, their lives possibly hanging in the balance.

I try not to make eye contact with waiting patients or their family members lest they plead to be seen now. Most just sit there in silence, their illnesses smouldering away. It's the noisy patients who grab the attention, the ones with agitation from acute mental health conditions, street drugs or some combination.

"Clifford, please stay calm." Tawny stares down a twenty-four-year-old man with acute alcohol intoxication.

"They're fucking trying to kill me," says Clifford.

Four uniformed Toronto police officers surround him. They're flanked by five uniformed hospital security officers.

"Cynthia, I need four-point restraints," says Tawny.

"Can I get a sedation order?" Cynthia asks.

"Twenty-five milligrams of loxapine and two milligrams of lorazepam," says Tawny.

"Fire, fire!" Molly's cries sound more urgent.

I make my way down a fairly narrow hall crammed with nine patients on stretchers accompanied by a smaller number of paramedics. In optimal times, patients who arrive by ambulance are offloaded to an ER stretcher and handed over to the nurses. When there are no available stretchers, as is the case today, the paramedics are in what's known as "offload delay" and by law must continue caring for their patients until the nurses can take over. A 2022 analysis of Ontario Health data by the *Toronto Star* found that offload times had nearly doubled in just three years.

"Somebody put out the fire!" Molly screams again.

I approach her stretcher. "I'm Dr. Goldman. Remember me?"

Molly utters a blood-curdling scream.

"Molly, what's wrong?" I try to focus my patient on the chief complaint.

"Please put out the fire." She momentarily looks right at me.

"What fire?" I ask.

"She's been saying that since we arrived," explains a paramedic named Virginia. "She was just moaning when we picked her up on the curb outside a shelter. She's thirty-six years old and has a history of polysubstance use, anxiety and schizophrenia. She vomited two times at the scene. We gave her Toradol for the pain but it's not helping."

I've seen Molly before, but I've never seen her this agitated.

Virginia uses her paramedic-issued equipment to monitor Molly's vitals. "Heart rate 126, respirations 22 with 97 per cent O_2 saturation on room air. Temp 37.2 deg C, and BP 96 over 62."

The elevated heart rate and lowish blood pressure could be signs of pneumonia or a kidney infection, or possibly even sepsis, a life-threatening condition that happens when the body's immune system has an extreme response to an infection. The reaction causes damage to the body's own tissues and organs. Molly's normal temperature makes an infection less likely, though not impossible.

"Put out the fire!" Molly emits a ninety-decibel scream directly into my ears.

"You keep talking about the fire." I hear myself sounding exasperated. "Where is the fire?"

"Fire over there." She raises her arm and points a finger towards a window near the ambulance bay.

Molly is in deep distress and nearly oblivious to me. I'm not connecting with her. Time wasted. Time that could be spent looking after patients who can describe their symptoms with precision. What doctors call "good historians."

I look in the general direction where Molly is pointing. That's when I see the alternating red and blue flashing lights of a parked ambulance. I point to the lights. "Is that what you mean by fire?" I ask Molly.

"Fire, fire!" she yells.

Virginia and I look at each other like we have the same thought at the same time. She radioes her partner. "Unit 8375, can you cut your emergency lights?"

The lights stop flashing. Instantly, Molly goes quiet.

And I calm down as well. Noise is a major distraction in ERs—loud conversations between healthcare providers and patients punctuated by even louder alarms and beeps. To me, the most annoying noise by far is the long, non-musical tone that precedes each intercom announcement.

"Beeeep. PSW to room 45."

"Beeeep. Service assistant to room 31."

"Beeeep. Pink-zone nurse pick up line 38."

Now that Molly is no longer screaming, I can focus more closely on her and her distress. I notice the furrowing of her brow and the tiny beads of sweat on her forehead. These are subtle but important physical signs of distress.

"Are you in pain?" I ask her. She doesn't reply. I listen to her heart and lungs, and then start pressing on her belly.

"Owwwwww!" she hollers and pushes my hand away.

Her abdomen is as rigid as a plank of wood and tender all over.

"Holy shit!" Virginia says. "Her belly was soft and non-tender when we picked her up outside the shelter."

"I believe you," I tell her. "Something's going on, and it's happening fast."

Tenderness in her belly means that Molly likely has peritonitis. It's a serious condition in which the lining of the abdomen, or the peritoneum, is acutely inflamed. There are many causes, but the most common is a burst appendix or an infection caused by a perforation or hole in the stomach or intestines.

Peritonitis is life-threatening and demands a prompt response. Some patients deteriorate so rapidly they need intensive care. Patients may also require surgery to deal with the source of the infection by removing the inflamed appendix or repairing the torn bowel. But before I ask the surgeons to see Molly, I have to confirm that she has a surgical condition. Generally, that means getting a CT scan of her belly. To get more detailed pictures, the radiologist may want to inject the patient with radiocontrast or dye by IV drip. Since radiocontrast can be toxic to the kidneys, we must first obtain blood work to make sure the kidneys have enough functional reserve to tolerate the dye.

When the ER is well staffed and has lots of beds, there's a great deal I can do to stabilize a patient like Molly. I can order bags of intravenous fluids to raise her blood pressure. I can use IV antibiotics to treat a suspected infection inside her belly. I can move her to the resuscitation room to receive one-on-one nursing.

Much earlier in my ER career, patients were routinely whisked inside the sliding doors and quickly placed onto stretchers. But that's no longer the norm. In some ERs, patients with serious and even life-threatening illnesses routinely wait six, eight or even ten hours just to be brought in. Some patients wait all day to be seen by an ER physician. Increasingly, some patients die waiting to be seen.

I strongly suspect Molly has something seriously wrong, but I can't wait for a stretcher to become available inside. I must figure out what's wrong with her here and now.

I rummage through the fanny pack on my belt and pull out an ultrasound probe with a long electrical cable.

Virginia's eyes get wide. "What are you doing?"

"A little high-tech magic," I say as I plug the cable into my phone. An app immediately pops up on my display. I tear open a small pack of ultrasound conducting gel and spread it on the probe.

"It's going to feel a bit cool and goopy," I tell Molly. I place the gooped-up probe on her right side where the lower ribs meet the uppermost part of her belly. Instantly, my phone shows a clear and crisp image of Molly's right kidney just underneath her liver, with an ominously large triangle-shaped black blob in between.

Virginia sees my expression and looks at the display. "What's that?" she asks.

"There's fluid in the belly," I tell her. "And a whole lot of it."

The peritoneal cavity normally contains a small amount of fluid that lubricates the tissues lining the abdominal wall and the walls of the vital organs. Molly's belly contains as much as a litre, if not two. But what kind of fluid is it? There are three possibilities, and each carries a very different prognosis. One is that it's a watery fluid called a transudate. This can be a sign of liver cirrhosis or heart failure; both are serious but not immediately life-threatening conditions.

The second type of fluid is pus caused by an infection from a perforated bowel or burst appendix. Infections like that can be lethal and often require surgery, but there's usually time to save the patient.

The third type of fluid is blood. If Molly has blood in her belly, it means there's a hemorrhage somewhere. The most common cause of acute bleeding inside the belly is trauma from being hit by a car or beaten badly. But there is no indication that Molly has been hit. From what I can see, there are no bruises on her abdomen.

Molly has started moaning softly.

The portable monitor sitting on her gurney says her heart rate has crept up to 132.

"What's Molly's BP?" I'm getting edgy as I wait for the paramedic to take her blood pressure.

"Ninety over forty-five," Virginia says with a tinge of alarm.

By itself, a blood pressure that's dropping slowly or a heart rate that's creeping up at a leisurely pace might not indicate anything life-threatening. But occurring together along with an ultrasound showing a belly full of fluid, they suggest a condition that's much more ominous.

"She's going into shock." I speak my thoughts out loud. As I've gotten older, I tend to do that more deliberately, so colleagues know I've still got it.

Hemorrhagic shock has four clinical stages, each with symptoms and signs that reflect a particular amount of blood loss and degree of danger. In class 1 shock, the acute blood loss is less than three-quarters of a litre. Patients in class 1 shock are slightly anxious but have normal heart rate and blood pressure. If you identify and control the source of bleeding, they're in no danger. Class 2 shock means acute blood loss of up to one and a half litres. Patients in this class have heart rates between 100 and 120 beats per minute, slightly increased respirations, slightly decreased blood pressure, cool, clammy skin and slight anxiety or agitation. Class 3 means up to two litres of acute blood loss. Patients in class 3 shock have heart rates greater than 120 beats per minute, increased respirations (often referred to as "air hunger"), decreased blood pressure and pronounced anxiety and confusion. Class 4 shock means more than two litres of blood loss. Patients in class 4 shock have very rapid heart rate, extremely rapid and shallow breathing, extremely low blood pressure, loss of consciousness, pale, cool skin and blue lips or fingernails.

Molly's symptoms and signs tell me she's going into class 3 shock. If I'm right, she's in grave danger. In the earliest stages of shock, the body compensates for blood loss by secreting shots of adrenaline that raise the heart and respiratory rates and narrow the arteries that supply less important organs such as the stomach and intestines. The adrenaline can keep Molly going for a while, but if we don't quickly identify the source of the bleeding and stop it, her shock will become irreversible and she will die.

"She could be bleeding to death," I tell Virginia, grabbing the foot end of the gurney. "We don't have a lot of time."

Virginia and I push Molly's stretcher towards the entrance to the ER.

"I think Molly's bleeding in her belly," I tell Cynthia, the team leader. "We need to bring her into resus now."

Resus isn't a playground for lower primates. It is shorthand for the resuscitation room.

Cynthia takes half a second to absorb the new challenge before swiping her key card in the security lock to open the door to the inside of the ER. "I'll let Lance and Rishna know you're on your way."

I just hope we can figure out why Molly is bleeding in time to save her.

Patients like Molly—those with an illness or injury who may be inching towards death in an ER waiting room—were once the exception. Nowadays there's often a Molly lurking in every overcrowded ER.

Dr. Raghu Venugopal is an emergency physician who works evening and overnight shifts at three busy ERs in downtown Toronto. He has lots of stories of finding the proverbial needle in the haystack—the one patient among dozens of very sick people who is actually closer than the others to dying.

Venugopal recalls one shift where he picked up the chart of a man in his twenties who was having chest pain. Our training and experience say that's nothing to worry about because young men don't get heart attacks. He went to see the man and immediately realized that, like Molly, he was going into shock in a hallway.

"He was dying in front of me," Venugopal told me, recalling the moment. Several life-threatening cardiac catastrophes flashed through his mind, the most lethal being an aortic dissection—a tear in the young man's aorta.

"Not on my watch," Venugopal thought. "We don't have a bed, but I don't care what anyone thinks. We're going to CT and then into the resuscitation room."

The CT scan showed that the young man's aorta was intact. Nevertheless, Venugopal and the paramedics took the patient to the resuscitation room. "And he suffers a cardiac arrest right there."

Venugopal, the nurses and the paramedics defibrillated the young man and brought him back. He was later found to have advanced coronary artery disease and needed an angioplasty to unblock his coronaries. He made a full recovery and has since gone back to work.

That man survived because of Venugopal's quick and decisive action, and because he had the time to recognize and save *his* Molly. But still, he worries that there may come a time when he has two or three Mollys to pull in at the same moment and won't know which one to choose.

The ER has always been a stressful place to work, but with near and actual misses happening with greater frequency, it's also becoming a scary place to work. One of the biggest and most far-reaching changes I've witnessed since I wrote *The Night Shift* is the impact of that fear and stress on the doctors, nurses and other healthcare providers who work alongside me. That includes paramedics like Virginia, who bring patients to the hospital. The lack of ER stretchers and the growing backlog of patients in the waiting room have meant that paramedics are unable to offload their patients and have to spend more and more hours—sometimes entire shifts—attending to people they have brought to the ER. Every hour they spend in the ER is an hour they cannot spend responding to emergencies in the field.

To deal with this problem, the Alberta government issued a guideline for paramedics to offload their patients to ER stretchers within forty-five minutes of arrival. How strictly that guideline has been followed is a matter of controversy.

As reported by CBC in early March 2023, the opposition NDP released an email it claimed was sent from a unit manager to ER staff at Calgary's Foothills Medical Centre. The email said that beginning on March 15, patients at Calgary ERs were to be offloaded by paramedics within forty-five minutes regardless of whether staff were available to care for them. "I know this comes as a big shock to all of us and I am not sure how we are going to manage this," the manager wrote. "Please know if there was anything I could do to prevent this I would but this is being mandated from the government." (The province denied that the guideline was an order. Kerry Williamson, a spokesperson for Alberta Health Services, said that forty-five minutes was a target, not a mandate.)

In September 2024, Athana Mentzelopoulos, then president and CEO of Alberta Health Services, sent a note to healthcare workers warning of increased ambulance calls during the fall and winter months. The note said a number of steps would be taken to address the issue, including increasing ER capacity and using the new ambulance offload guideline. It stated that when the system was at critical capacity and few or no ambulances were available, paramedics could be released to respond to calls rather than waiting in the ER with their patients.

Dr. Paul Parks is an ER physician at Medicine Hat Regional Hospital in Alberta, and a past president of the Alberta Medical Association. He told me that the offload policy was implemented with no corresponding increase in nurses, doctors or stretchers. It's his view that the policy has had at least two unintended consequences. The first is to privilege patients who arrive by ambulance over those who come in on their own by putting the ambulance patients on ER stretchers sooner, even though, perhaps counterintuitively, it's not uncommon for people who bring themselves to the ER to be sicker and in more urgent need of care than patients brought in by paramedics.

The second unintended consequence is to force nurses to be redeployed from rooms inside the ER to the offload hallways to care for patients on offload stretchers. "We have them go work in the hallway for the offloaded patients who still haven't gotten into the emergency department proper," said Parks. He told me that sometimes the demand to redeploy nurses to the waiting room is so extreme that the ER must close beds on the inside. "It's caused us some really perverse, ironic struggles. You take your good ER nurses that want to be doing emergency nursing in the actual ER, but there they are in a hallway with eight or ten patients."

Increasingly, nurses have given up trying to effect change and instead are quitting the ER altogether. Hospitals across Canada are reporting high nurse vacancy rates. A report by Ontario's acting auditor general, for example, found that at some hospitals in the province, as many as one in four nursing jobs across all departments are unfilled. At William Osler Health System, which runs hospitals in Brampton and Etobicoke, the nurse vacancy rate jumped from 6 per cent in 2019–20 to 26 per cent in 2022–23. During the same period, the vacancy rate at Toronto's Hospital for Sick Children (SickKids) climbed from 8 per cent to 22 per cent. Other provinces are faring worse. At the beginning of 2023, Nova Scotia Health reported that eighteen units at regional hospitals had a nurse vacancy rate of 50 per cent or more. The ER at the Cape Breton Regional Hospital had an astronomically high 80 per cent vacancy rate of licensed practical nurses.

Some of this was caused by the Covid pandemic, but some is a result of the increasingly stressful work environment—nurses in frantically busy ERs routinely miss breaks and are often compelled to work overtime to cover for colleagues who call in sick. Some nurses are also going to the United States, where pay and benefits are better. That may have changed with the Trump administration's new and more hostile attitude towards Canada.

And it's not just nurses who are quitting. More recently, ER physicians have started heading for the exits as well. Dr. Michael Howlett, president of the Canadian Association of Emergency

Physicians, or CAEP, told *Maclean's* in 2024 that colleagues across Canada are giving up the ER to work in walk-in clinics that are still stressful but have more predictable hours, or are taking on teaching and administrative roles in hospitals. The result is a large and growing shortfall of ER physicians. "CAEP predicts that we're going to have a lack of 1,500 emergency physicians in Canada by 2025," said Howlett. "That number is going to keep growing." Nothing has changed in the meantime to alter that prediction.

Beyond the regular ER physicians who are quitting, there's a new and disturbing trend: The chiefs and heads of departments are also packing it in. When Dr. Carolyn Snider finished her first five-year term as chief of the emergency department at St. Michael's Hospital in Toronto, she chose not to re-up for a second term.

"I have a moral responsibility as a leader," Snider said, "and was responsible for dealing with every critical incident and every patient relation related to things I had no agency to change. And that is why it is so hard to be a leader in emergency medicine . . . More and more leaders are stepping down before the end of their terms because the systems aren't allowing for the match between agency and accountability."

Shortfalls of doctors and nurses in urban ERs lead to scheduling snafus and overworked frontline staff. Burnout is a constant threat, and thoughts of quitting are ever present. And we're not only talking about people who've been in the field for decades. In January 2022, Jacelyn Wingerter, a registered nurse with less than a year of experience in the ER at Saskatoon's Royal University Hospital, told CBC that she already felt defeated. "You don't get a break. You have to run for 12 hours straight doing one thing after another."

In smaller rural and more remote hospitals, those shortfalls sometimes force ERs to close for anywhere from half a day to several weeks. When *The Night Shift* was published, ER closures almost never happened. Fifteen years later, they have become a regular occurrence in many parts of Canada.

My friend and colleague Dr. Ken Milne has called the ER the light in the lighthouse that never goes out, no matter what. But in a growing number of ERs in almost every province and territory, the light is flickering. Increasingly, people on the front lines talk openly about the "collapse" of emergency medicine. In 2024, CAEP published *EM:POWER: The Future of Emergency Care*, a 328-page report on the crisis in the country's ERs and what to do about it. "Nurses and physicians show extreme levels of burnout," the report noted, "and are quitting in alarming numbers; ambulance offload delays are soaring, and patients are leaving emergency departments without care and with limited recourse."

Dr. Steve Flindall has worked at a busy suburban Toronto ER for twenty-one years, and he has seen everything the CAEP report described and more. "Every time I think we're on the verge of collapse, people just seem to step up," he told me. "The emergency staff just keep doing more with less, and despite that, we make space and give care. But I don't know how much extra we've got to give."

Dr. Raghu Venugopal sees things in terms of accountability metrics: Patients waiting longer than recommended to be triaged. Kids waiting twelve hours or more for fairly minor complaints like allergic reactions. Admitted patients waiting hours or even days to get a hospital bed. "If we look at multiple indicators," he said, "the emergency room system in Canada has collapsed."

All this means that the margin of error to save patients like Molly gets smaller and smaller.

7:30 p.m.

"Service assistant to room 60 stat." Cynthia's voice on the intercom sounds calm but purposeful.

Molly's moans fill the air as Virginia and I push her stretcher through the sliding doors of room 60, the resuscitation room. This fully equipped suite has almost everything we need to save her life. Lance and Rishna, the nurses working the resuscitation area, have just started their twelve-hour night shift. They're already priming IVs and gathering medications.

"Two fourteen-gauge IVs running wide open with Ringer's lactate," I tell Lance. Ringer's lactate is an intravenous fluid we administer to replace lost electrolytes and fluids in patients who are dehydrated or in shock.

Virginia and I slide Molly's paramedic stretcher alongside the gurney in the centre of the room.

Tawny walks briskly into the room. "Can I help?" She's followed by Cynthia.

"Let's get Molly on the gurney on three." I grab the orange paramedic blanket underneath Molly at the foot of the stretcher. Tawny moves to the head of the stretcher, and Virginia and Cynthia take the sides. "One, two, three."

Molly moans loudly as we slide her onto the gurney.

"I'll take the airway," says Tawny. She preps to do a rapid sequence intubation so she can intubate Molly in a hurry. "Get me a hundred milligrams of ketamine and sixty of rocuronium," she calls out to Rishna. Ketamine is a powerful sedative and rocuronium is a muscle relaxant. "And call the respiratory therapist to grab the video laryngoscope."

More nurses join the gathering team to save Molly.

Lance has already collected tubes so he can get blood work and insert the IV with one poke. "Do you want a trauma panel?" he asks me. A trauma panel is a group of standard blood tests ordered on trauma patients: a complete blood count, electrolytes, creatinine, amylase, coagulation screen, blood alcohol level, venous blood gases, lactate level and a blood group and screen.

"Affirmative to that," I say, "plus type and cross for four units of packed red blood cells. Molly has an acute abdomen and a whole lot of free fluid. It could be pus but I'm pretty sure she's bleeding." And then I add, "Get an HCG stat. And get a service assistant to run the blood work up to the lab."

The HCG, or human chorionic gonadotropin, is a pregnancy blood test. Because Molly is a thirty-six-year-old and (I assume) of child-bearing potential, it's essential to find out if she's pregnant.

Cynthia and another nurse, Jason, put adhesive ECG leads on Molly's chest and extremities. "Cycling BP every two minutes," says Cynthia.

"Brian, how much TXA do you want?" Rishna is drawing up tranexamic acid into a syringe. This is a medication that binds to a receptor on a protein named plasminogen, found in blood plasma. Plasminogen plays an essential role in dissolving blood clots. By blocking the receptor, TXA helps slow down the rate of bleeding by coaxing Molly's blood to clot.

"Two grams, please."

Rishna pushes the dose.

Meanwhile, a respiratory therapist named Rebecca wheels a video laryngoscope up to Tawny at the head of the bed. "What size tube do you want?" she asks.

"Seven point five," Tawny replies. "Molly, we're going to give you some medication to make you sleepy, and then I'm going to put a tube into your throat so you can breathe easier."

"Shall I push the ketamine now?" Lance asks.

"Yes," Tawny replies. "Then wait one minute before giving the rocuronium."

The sequence of medications is deliberate. If you're paralyzing a patient with rocuronium, you don't want her to be awake for that, because the experience is extremely traumatic. So the ketamine is administered first, and Tawny waits about a minute for the sedation to kick in.

Ninety seconds later, Molly is no longer moaning. But since her muscles are completely paralyzed, she isn't breathing either.

Tawny looks into Molly's mouth as she inserts the video laryngoscope. Rebecca turns on the video screen, which shows a perfect view of the inside of Molly's oral cavity. Tawny looks at the screen and can see exactly where she's going as she advances the scope over Molly's tongue and towards her epiglottis. "I see the vocal cords," she says matter-of-factly.

Rebecca hands Tawny a 7.5 millimetre endotracheal tube with a bendable stylet inside.

Tawny continues to look at the screen as she passes the tube through the vocal cords. "I'm in," she says. She removes the stylet and holds the precious breathing tube in place as Rebecca quickly attaches a sensor to track Molly's carbon dioxide level and connects the sensor wire to the monitor.

"I'll start setting up the ventilator," Rebecca says.

"Rishna, start a ketamine drip at fifteen milligrams per hour and titrate," says Tawny. The drip will keep Molly sedated for as long as she is intubated and on a ventilator.

Suddenly, the blood pressure alarm on the vital signs monitor starts chiming. The systolic blood pressure, which was 90 millimetres of mercury just a few minutes ago, is now 75.

"What dose of Levophed do you want?" Cynthia is two steps ahead of me. She's already preparing an infusion of norepinephrine bitartrate, a vasoconstrictor. Levophed is a go-to medication that raises the blood pressure. It's essential for patients in shock.

"Start at twenty micrograms per minute and taper to maintain a systolic pressure of ninety," I reply.

"Resus nurse, stat result on line 38," says Vivica over the intercom.

Rishna and Lance are occupied, so Cynthia picks up the phone. Everybody keeps an eye on the team leader, who scribbles figures onto a scratchpad and gives her last name to the lab technician on the line before hanging up.

"Hemoglobin is seventy-two," says Cynthia. "Lactate six point seven. The HCG is positive."

The positive HCG is the missing piece of the puzzle. It means that Molly is pregnant.

That fact almost guarantees that the fluid in her belly is blood. The most likely explanation for the blood is that she has an ectopic pregnancy that grew through one of her fallopian tubes until it ripped the tube apart and started to bleed like a firehose into her belly cavity.

You might think it would have been simpler and saved valuable time had I been able to see the ectopic pregnancy when I put my ultrasound probe on Molly's belly in the hallway. Seeing a live pregnancy in the belly would have nailed the diagnosis. But by the time the fallopian tube ruptures, there may not be any pregnancy left to see on an ultrasound. Most often, an ectopic pregnancy is assumed when the HCG is positive and the womb is found on ultrasound to be empty.

"Two units of O-negative blood," I call out. O negative is the universal donor blood type. It's the kind of blood we keep in a fridge in the ER for those occasions when a patient is so gravely ill that she needs a transfusion before the blood bank can determine her actual blood type. O negative is used most often in cases of trauma and any other occurrence of hemorrhage when the blood type is unknown.

"Sounds like a job for the rapid infuser," says a colleague nicknamed Fix as he walks into the room pushing an IV pole with a device shaped like a rectangular box mounted in the middle. An ER resident named Shirley and a nurse named Christine follow close behind. The rapid infuser is a device that warms and delivers extremely large volumes of blood products and intravenous fluids.

When a patient has a rapid and uncontrolled hemorrhage, like Molly does, the rapid infuser is a lifesaver.

Fix's first name is Philip. He got the nickname because he knows how every medical device in the ER works. And if it's broken, he knows how to fix it. He and Shirley started at noon today. They are currently assigned to the ambulatory zone, or AZ, of the ER, where they've been seeing patients with relatively minor conditions such as cuts and ankle sprains.

Nearly eight hours into their day, they should be exhausted, but Fix doesn't show it. He exudes boundless energy as he works with Christine to set up the rapid infuser, all the while teaching Shirley so that she'll be able to set it up herself next time.

"Thanks for stepping in, Fix," I tell him. "You too, Tawny."

"Teamwork makes the dream work," says Fix.

"Cynthia, can you have Vivica page OBGYN stat?"

7:45 p.m.

After two units of blood, Molly's blood pressure is 100 over 45 and her heart rate is 105. She's still in pain, but she appears more stable.

Soming, a senior resident in obstetrics and gynecology, and Ben, a second-year OBGYN resident, are seeing her in the resuscitation room. A service assistant arrives to help the two doctors and Rishna transport Molly to the operating room, where they'll remove her ruptured fallopian tube and repair whatever damage they find inside.

"Good save, Dr. Goldman," says Soming, who at twenty-eight is young enough to be my daughter. When I was her age and just starting out, I wanted to be called Dr. Goldman. Now that I'm close to retirement, I wish younger docs still called me Brian.

"The team did an amazing job," I reply, deflecting the accolade to its proper place.

All told, six nurses, three attending ER doctors, two learners and one respiratory therapist converged on room 60 to save Molly's life. That's a good chunk of the resources and personnel of the ER. In the interim, nine more patients arrived in the waiting room.

Cynthia and I glance uneasily at one another as we walk back to the triage area.

"That could have been a disaster," she whispers.

Cynthia is right. Molly's ruptured ectopic pregnancy started with a trickle of blood in her belly that grew over who knows how many hours or even days.

I start to play "what if" in my mind. What if I didn't see Molly before everyone else? What if I didn't listen to Cynthia, who was just trying to deal with the noise Molly was making? What if I didn't have my ultrasound probe with me? What if I didn't pull her stretcher into the ER?

Molly is on her way to the operating room. She has a good chance of surviving in part because we got lucky and found the needle in the haystack—the one patient out of dozens in the waiting room who could wait no longer.

It's not even 8:00 p.m. My actual casino shift doesn't begin for another hour. It's going to be a long night. I can feel it.

CHAPTER TWO

WAITING ROOM

8:00 p.m.

"I hear you started without me." Ahu, a second-year resident in family medicine, approaches me in the triage bay wearing a big grin.

"I got called in early," I reply while looking at the list of patients waiting to be seen. "I thought about calling you in too but got sidetracked by a patient."

"You should have called me." She sounds disappointed at missing out on a great learning opportunity. It's how I would have reacted when I was a resident.

"Sorry about that." By way of explanation, I point to the throng of patients in the waiting room.

For Ahu's one-month rotation in the ER, I'm her supervisor. Next year, she'll be doing an extra year of training to become an ER specialist. In her first year of residency, Ahu did a mandatory two-month rotation in the ER. In this, her second year, she has several months of elective, or non-compulsory, rotations. Residents use these slots to gather additional experience in areas of medicine where they feel the passion to learn more.

But there's also a tactical reason for putting in extra time in the

ER. Spending her elective time here is a great way to show her commitment.

I'm really glad she's on this evening. We've worked together three times, and I'm impressed by her knowledge and her poise.

"There's plenty more patients to see." I look out at the slew of patients in the waiting room. "There's a couple of people waiting to be seen inside. You look in on them, and I'll try to slog through what's stacking up out here."

"We'll catch up, Dr. Goldman," she says to me. "Did I ever tell you that Ahu means 'gazelle' in Persian?"

That makes me smile.

Like all other scheduled ER shifts, the casino shift has a particular order of duties. As the freshest doctor on duty, I will see the most acutely ill patients for the next two hours, until the night shift doctor arrives. Tawny, the ER doc who preceded me, moves over to the rapid assessment zone, where she'll typically see patients with chest or abdominal pain, pregnancy-related bleeding or gynecological problems. Fix returns to the ambulatory care zone, where he's seeing patients with minor issues like cuts and lacerations, burns, earaches and bone fractures.

With no empty stretchers available inside the ER, the waiting room is my examining room. I scan the packed space looking for a patient named Larry. The place is buzzing with even more patients than when I first got here. Zahir, a sixty-two-year-old man who lives on the street, is slumped on the seat of his walker. Tawny's patient Clifford, now sedated, has been placed on a stretcher.

"Larry?" I call out, looking for a spark of recognition. Patients not named Larry and their loved ones try to grab my attention instead. Given how long they've been waiting, I can't blame them.

Healthcare providers believe that the saying about the squeaky wheel getting the grease was coined with patients in mind. Not infrequently, the quiet ones are the sickest.

Out of the corner of my eye, I spot the hand of an older woman waving weakly.

"I'm Dr. Goldman," I say, taking in Larry's tired and sunken eyes. He's ninety-one years old and looks dehydrated and debilitated. He registered to be seen at 4:20 p.m., more than three and a half hours ago.

"He probably can't hear you in all this noise," says the woman. "He's hard of hearing. I'm his wife, Helen."

"Pleased to meet you, Helen and Larry," I reply. "Come with me."

Helen appears just slightly more robust than her husband. She grabs a bag while helping Larry slowly get up from his chair.

"Can I carry something for you?" I'm trying to be solicitous, but I'm also trying to speed things up. Every minute saved is a minute I spend seeing the next patient.

"We'll manage," says Helen. More often than not, no matter how ill they are, patients and their loved ones refuse offers of help.

Larry's shuffling gait makes me suspect he has Parkinson's disease. He holds his belly as he walks, grimacing as the two follow me on the short journey to a large room just off the waiting area. It contains four stretchers separated by privacy curtains. We shuttle patients in and out of this room to do quick assessments, ECGs and blood work.

I help Larry climb onto the only unoccupied stretcher. He's not unstable like Molly. His heart rate and blood pressure are okay. But he has a slight fever and he looks ill.

"What's going on, Larry?" I ask in a loud and deliberate voice. It's less noisy here than in the open waiting room. Still, there are close conversations happening on either side of us, and I'm hoping my patient can hear me.

Larry has a puzzled look on his face.

"Tell the doctor what's wrong," says Helen.

"My belly hurts," he replies instantly. "I keep throwing up. I can't hold anything down."

"I guess your lips are harder to read than mine," says Helen, a tiny smile forming at the corners of her mouth.

"How long have the two of you been married?" I ask Helen.

"Seventy years this June," she says.

"That's beautiful," I reply. "How many kids do you have?"

"We had one son," says Helen. "He died of leukemia when he was four."

"I'm so sorry to hear that."

"It was a long time ago." Helen looks off into the distance.

"I need to feel your belly," I tell Larry. "Helen, can you ask him to point to where it hurts?"

The abdomen is divided into four quadrants that are bisected by the belly button. Larry points to his left lower quadrant. I press methodically on each of the other three quadrants before zeroing in on the area that hurts.

"Owwww," says Larry as I find the tender spot and something else: a mass of tissue that feels as hard as a rock.

"How long has he had pain?" I ask Helen.

"At least six months, maybe longer," she sighs. "I tried to get him to see the doctor, but he refused."

You don't need to be an astute physician to know that a tender abdomen and a hard mass likely mean cancer. Judging by the look on Helen's face, you don't need to be a physician at all.

"Larry, something's going on in your belly. We need to get a CT scan to see what it is. You're also dehydrated, and I want to start an intravenous so I can give you some fluids. To make you more comfortable, I'd like to give you something for the pain and something for the nausea."

"I'm right beside you, dear," says Helen.

Larry looks more comfortable relaxing on the stretcher in the side room. I gather myself for what I need to do next.

"I hate to do this, but I have to ask you and Helen to go back to the waiting area and take a seat. We'll try to get you in as soon as we can."

As I rush back to the triage area to scribble some notes and write some orders, Larry and Helen make their way back to the same chairs where I found them. Most people do that.

"Cynthia, I need blood work on Larry so I can prep him for a CT scan of his abdomen." I make sure I sound like I'm asking her and not issuing an order. "I know you're short-staffed out here, but I'm hoping he can get a stretcher inside."

"That's not going to happen until they do something about the bed situation upstairs. We can do the blood work and maybe start an IV."

"He's in a lot of pain. Can we get him some hydromorphone?"

"Just write the order," Cynthia sighs quietly. "We'll get to it when we can."

"I know you will."

I know that Cynthia is as distressed about any delay in providing pain relief to Larry as I am about making him sit in a crowded waiting room when he needs to rest.

At this moment, there's not much either of us can do about it.

The upsetting thing is that patients like Larry are no longer exceptional. "Hallway medicine" has long defined the crisis in Canada's ERs. The term has been around since at least 1952, when journalist Sidney Katz began to write articles on the state of healthcare in this country prior to the federal Medical Care Act. This legislation, which was passed in 1966, provided payment for half of provincial and territorial costs for medical services provided by doctors. In his articles, Katz gave accounts of patients being cared for "on kitchen floors before being transferred to corridors." Those kitchen floors were the forerunner of the hallways of today.

What's new is that ER care has shifted to the waiting room. Dr. Catherine Varner is an ER colleague of mine in Toronto. As deputy editor of the *Canadian Medical Association Journal*, she's a keen observer and chronicler of the deteriorating state of the ER system. Calling waiting room medicine a "new field," Varner says that providers are being forced to adapt to seeing patients on chairs in the waiting room instead of on stretchers inside the ER or even in an ambulance parked on the hospital driveway. "There have been times over the last two years where I'm standing in our waiting room with many patients waiting to be seen—many of whom are uncomfortable and sick—where you want to sort of shout from the rooftops and say, 'This is what a health-care system in collapse looks like,'" says Varner.

Dr. Raghu Venugopal, who works at three ERs in Toronto, told me that he regularly cares for waiting room patients. "I had a patient in their nineties with a bowel perforation in a chair [in the waiting room]," he recalled. "I had a patient over age ninety with an intracranial hemorrhage and a spinal fracture. Mind you, the spinal fracture was stable, [but] that patient had to wait in a chair."

This isn't something unique to Toronto. Seeing and treating patients seated in the waiting room is happening at ERs across Canada.

"On my last shift, I had a young woman who came in with what she thought was a miscarriage," said Dr. Lorri Beatty, an ER physician at the Halifax Infirmary. "She ended up completing her entire miscarriage in the waiting room while she waited six hours to get in and see us. I feel like I start just about every interaction now with, 'I'm so sorry it's taken me this long to see you.'"

Beatty is apologizing for the wait to be seen, but increasingly, we also have to apologize for *where* people are being seen.

Venugopal told me with some amazement that most patients he sees don't complain when they are asked to return to the waiting room, as Larry was. "I think people are a little bit shocked," he said. "But because of the authority we bring to our job, ninety per cent will comply because they see the environmental situation."

He feels even more distraught when he has patients who are so sick they can't stay upright in a chair. "I was called by security to go see someone on the floor," he recalled. "I came across an elderly [man] who was lying on the floor in the waiting room and who was awaiting admission to hospital under internal medicine. The patient had multiple reasons for being in the hospital. And I asked him, 'Sir, are you okay? Are you injured? Why are you on the floor?' He said, 'Doctor, I'm sick and I'm tired and I have to lie down.'"

This man wasn't Venugopal's only patient who has needed to recline in an ER with no available stretchers. The doctor's voice rose as he talked to me about these people. "I feel rage," he said. "I feel rage that the system and I could treat a senior citizen this way. I feel that incredible disrespect that we are conveying to someone at that point in their life. They're calling for help and this is what we offer."

Some of the worst stories I've heard of being forced to care for sick patients on chairs and on floors in the waiting room have come from Alberta.

Dr. Paul Parks has been working in the province since 2000 and is now at the Medicine Hat Regional Hospital after nine years in Edmonton. The hospital is the designated regional trauma centre. It has an ER that operates twenty-four hours a day and also provides acute care, intensive and neonatal intensive care, kidney care, cardio-respiratory services and more.

As mentioned, Parks has been active in provincial medical politics. He has been with the Alberta Medical Association (AMA) since 2007 and served as president in 2023–24. In that role, he heard from many distressed colleagues across the province. One ER doc, for example, told him about a patient who'd suffered an acute stroke and was paralyzed on one side of the body but still had to wait twelve hours to be seen. Because he wasn't able to walk, his family members had to carry him to the bathroom and back.

"I don't think your average Canadians and Albertans can really imagine what it would be like to be with your loved one with a stroke for twelve hours," Parks told me. "And you can't get inside the ER and you can't get them care."

Parks said that Alberta ER doctors have also seen pregnant women miscarry in the waiting room, as Lorri Beatty did in Halifax. (Twenty-first-century MDs can do a lot of things, but they can't stop a miscarriage in progress.) "You never would have thought that you'd be talking to a twenty-five-year-old mom having a miscarriage," he said, "[and] having this conversation with them in the waiting room, where everybody can hear and there's no sense of privacy or dignity."

In 2023, Parks heard of a case involving a sixteen-year-old girl with abdominal pain who was diagnosed with appendicitis. She needed an operation and had to be transferred to another hospital to get it. Even though the receiving hospital had accepted her, it was so busy there that the girl still waited at least twelve hours to be seen. Before she could even get to the operating room, her appendix burst.

The risk of rupture, or perforation, to the appendix increases the longer appendicitis treatment is delayed. Most cases of a ruptured appendix occur between forty-eight and seventy-two hours after the onset of symptoms, so in this case the delay in surgery was a factor in the development of perforation. A ruptured appendix is considered an emergency. It releases bacteria into the abdomen, and if left untreated, it leads to complications that include widespread infection inside the belly, abscess, sepsis and even death.

"She's young and healthy, so thankfully she didn't die," said Parks. "Thankfully she didn't get septic complications. But I guarantee you her clinical care and outcome were significantly impacted because of [the delay in treatment]."

Others have not been so lucky. In January 2022, CTV News reported that a person had died while waiting for a bed inside the Red Deer Regional Hospital Centre. According to a spokesperson for Alberta Health Services, "The patient had been triaged, and later reassessed by emergency department staff, and was waiting for further care in an emergency department space."

"I've seen cases where patients have been in the waiting room and then they code," said Parks, using medical jargon for a cardiac arrest. Despite doctors' best efforts to resuscitate them, some of those people died. Parks noted that often those patients were frail seniors who were severely ill with conditions like chronic heart, lung and kidney disease, and their deaths would not have been entirely unexpected. But he also knows of cases where people younger and otherwise healthier have deteriorated unexpectedly in the waiting room and might not have had they been seen sooner.

"There was a case about a four-month-old that went into respiratory arrest because they had RSV bronchiolitis and we couldn't get them in," Parks told me. RSV is short for respiratory syncytial virus, a common respiratory illness that usually produces cold-like symptoms such as a runny nose and mild fever. In infants, however, it can result in a more severe condition called bronchiolitis, which causes swelling and irritation and a build-up of mucus in the small airways of the lungs. Infants have immature lungs, and when they develop bronchiolitis, they are more likely to need hospitalization. During the winters of 2022–23 and 2023–24, big increases in RSV infections among infants led to a spike in hospital admissions across the country.

"A four-month-old with severe bronchiolitis due to RSV is not someone who should be waiting in the waiting room," noted Parks. "But that's kind of the reality of examples we're talking about." In this case, the sick baby and the parents remained in the waiting room for hours because there were no spaces available inside the ER. When the baby stopped breathing, nurses and doctors wheeled them into a non-clinical "quiet room" usually reserved for families dealing with the emotional aftermath of a death or a life-limiting diagnosis. Parks said that the baby was intubated quickly and survived. But that's not the point. "I think the average person out there would think our healthcare system can rapidly take care of our kids and younger people, right?"

Anecdotally speaking, Dr. Parks told me that at hospitals across Alberta, the number of admitted patients in ERs waiting for beds on the wards upstairs may be far higher than generally reported.

"It's usually in the neighbourhood of a hundred per cent of what bed capacity [in the ER] could be," he said. "If you've got fifty beds, you've got fifty, sixty, seventy patients in the waiting room. In the smaller regional hospitals, where you have twenty-five to thirty beds, they'll often have thirty, forty or fifty patients in the waiting room. This becomes this normalization of deviant care. It's just so suboptimal, the conditions that we are frequently dealing with."

I admire ER doctors like Paul Parks and Raghu Venugopal

because they push back against the idea of caring for patients in "deviant" locations. I recall how weird it felt the first time I did a physical on someone lying on a gurney in a waiting room packed with patients and their families. Now I hardly even notice, and I know many of my colleagues feel the same. We just attend to the patient as if waiting room medicine is simply part of the job.

But this *shouldn't* be normal. It's injurious to patients because waiting rooms do not offer privacy, dignity, comfort or even the tools of the trade found beyond the sliding doors. I'm glad that I was able to diagnose Molly because I had a portable ultrasound I could whip out of my fanny pack and place on her abdomen. But I'm also conscious of the fact that the same corridor where I diagnosed her doesn't have, say, a heart monitor or a blood pressure machine. I'm not the only ER physician who feels this way.

"We signed up to take care of people, and we're currently trying to practise medicine where you can't take good care of people," said Dr. Amy Nason, an ER physician in Halifax. "What if I'm the one who makes a critical error while I'm trying to take care of people, not in the right spaces with not the right equipment and not the right staffing ratios, and I lose my job and I lose my livelihood? And what if I am the one to hurt somebody because I just can't see what's going on with him or I can't take care of what's going on with him with what I have available to me right now?"

In many provinces, ER physicians are dealing with these issues for the first time. But in Alberta, there is a sense of déjà vu. Back in the late 1990s and early 2000s, the province struggled to cope with severe emergency department overcrowding in the wake of several hospital closures and large cuts to the capacity of the healthcare system. The province was able to claw its way back in the early 2010s after Alberta Health Services spearheaded several initiatives designed to address wait times and overcrowding. AHS also created more hospital and long-term care beds and established maximum wait times to be seen in the ER. But then ground was lost again because of problems that ERs across Canada face, such as an aging population.

At the turn of this century, just under 13 per cent of Canadians were seniors. By 2022, that figure had risen to nearly 19 per cent. And the people we see in the ER aren't just older; their illnesses tend to be much more complex.

These issues have led to increased demand for medical services, but there has been little corresponding increase in long-term and acute care bed capacity. "The last hospital built in the Edmonton Zone was [in] 1988," Parks told me. "Since then, the population for that zone has at least doubled!"

The strains are being felt across the entire healthcare system, but the ER is still seen as the safety valve for shortcomings elsewhere. "Everything is directed to the ER now," Parks noted. "Surgical delays, cancer treatment delays, mental health access block, no primary care, you name it—go to the ER."

It's a problem that can't be fixed, Parks said, with baby steps and little sprinkles of money here and there. "It's going to take some very large leaps and substantial changes in how we deliver health and how we invest in it." The first step, he told me, is for the provinces to admit there's a crisis, meet with stakeholders and make long-term investments in wellness and primary care. That would help patients get the treatments they need without having to go to the ER. The solution, he said, does not lie in "tweaking funding from political cycle to cycle."

I asked Parks if he had faith that Alberta's current government would address the ER crisis.

"Honestly, I'm not sure on this one," he said. "The hole has gotten very deep. Of course, you have to have hope. I wouldn't have taken on the massive role of being the president of the AMA if I thought it was totally hopeless."

There's another anxiety-provoking aspect to waiting room medicine. Some patients are so disturbed by the wait (not to mention the spectacle) that they leave the emergency department before seeing a healthcare provider. Hospitals and ER physicians like me know a lot about these patients. We even have a name for them. We designate these would-be patients as "LWBS," which stands for "left without being seen."

In some ways, it may be tempting to dismiss LWBS patients from one's mind. But those of us who work in the ER maintain a healthy concern lest the patient who departs the hospital before being assessed by the physician on duty harbours a life-threatening ailment.

On the evening of December 4, 2024, thirty-nine-year-old Adam Burgoyne had chest pain and shortness of breath. Burgoyne, who was living in Montreal and worked at RBC as a senior manager of software development, was taken by ambulance to the ER at the Centre hospitalier de l'Université de Montréal, commonly called CHUM. En route, paramedics gave him ASA and nitroglycerin.

At triage, Burgoyne's vital signs were found to be normal and an ECG did not show a heart attack. Burgoyne was given a priority 3 score, which indicates that his condition was deemed not to be urgent. He was sent to a waiting room, where he remained for six hours without further evaluation.

In the early hours of December 5, unwilling to wait longer, Burgoyne left the ER and went home. According to his obituary, he died the next day. The cause of death was an aortic dissection, in which a rip in his aorta caused him to bleed to death internally.

We know all of this for several reasons. First, the case was investigated by the province's coroner's office, which launched an investigation ten days after Burgoyne's death.

The second reason why Burgoyne's case is so well known is that on December 5, Burgoyne himself posted on X about his long wait to be seen and his decision to leave the ER. Since then, and likely because of his death, that post has been viewed nearly 23 million times as of early June 2025 and has generated more than 1,800 replies, including one from X owner Elon Musk, who wrote, "Wow, sorry to hear that. Life is fragile."

For decades, ERs have been cataloguing LWBS patients. In the years before Covid, studies showed that between 2.5 and 4.8 per cent of patients left Canadian ERs without seeing a doctor. In the US, the national benchmark for LWBS is one per cent of patients, and the national average has climbed between 1.1 and 2.1 per cent between January 2017 and December 2021. Some hospitals have rates of 10 per cent and higher.

An Ontario study published in 2024 in *JACEP Open*, the journal of the American College of Emergency Physicians, found that as many as 5.7 per cent of patients were classified as LWBS. Compared with the years before Covid, those who left without being seen during the 2022–23 fiscal year had a significantly higher rate of being hospitalized or dying in the seven days after leaving the ER. The study's authors concluded, "Our findings are an important signal of possible deterioration in overall quality of care within a large universal healthcare system, with the potential for severe consequences for patients."

In the report of her investigation into Adam Burgoyne's death, coroner Géhane Kamel referred to his long wait to be seen and the resulting aborted visit to the ER as "rather an alarming situation." In her report (translated from French), she wondered if it would not have been "more judicious" for the triage nurses at CHUM to assign Burgoyne a priority 2 designation, indicating a greater degree of clinical urgency. Burgoyne would then have been assigned a stretcher instead of being sent back to the waiting room. Had he been assessed and attended to sooner, it's possible that Burgoyne might not have left the ER. The coroner also wondered whether the decreased number of medical staff on duty at night played a role in Burgoyne's six-hour wait to be seen.

Coroners do not assign fault. In this case, the coroner issued recommendations to the provincial physician and nursing regulatory authorities—the Collège des médecins du Québec and the Ordre des infirmières et infirmiers du Québec—to review the procedures used at CHUM to ensure they met professional standards. She noted that the hospital cooperated fully in her investigation.

For its part, the hospital said in a statement to the *Montreal Gazette* that it had updated its training for triage nurses, provided clearer definitions for chest pain symptoms, implemented mandatory reassessments for patients in the waiting room and increased staffing levels on night shifts. "Since the beginning of the process, the CHUM has collaborated fully with the coroner's office," a hospital spokesperson told the *Gazette*. "Providing safe, quality care to all patients is a priority for the CHUM. Out of respect for the confidentiality of the files, we will not comment further."

The hospital has taken sensible, prudent measures to try to prevent patients who have potentially serious causes of chest pain from leaving the ER without being seen. But no rule can't at times be bent, if not broken, when circumstances and an overloaded system lead to intolerable waits.

8:35 p.m.

Across the waiting room, Larry is still sitting in a chair, thirty-five minutes after I first saw him, more than four hours since he arrived in the ER. He looks exhausted. I'm glad he now has an IV catheter taped to the back of his left forearm. I hope that a dose of hydromorphone will control his pain. I watch as a service assistant comes to take him to the CT room. She helps Larry up from his chair and motions him to follow her. Larry hangs on to his IV pole like it's a rollator. Helen follows closely behind. She meets my eyes as they walk slowly through the glass door and into the ER.

Seeing Helen and Larry reminds me of something poignant that Dr. Raghu Venugopal said about waiting room medicine. "You and I both know we can provide a lot of care in a chair. But when you're sick and feeling unwell, to be attended to in a bed means someone is tending to your illness, someone gives a damn, and someone wants to relieve the suffering."

In medicine, the currency of professionalism is clinical competence. Venugopal is a whiz at emergency medicine. But he's also its conscience. And he believes that waiting room medicine signals that we've lost something important.

"The watchword for me is decency," he told me. "I say we have become flagrantly indecent. I'm going to suggest that the simplest, [most] low cost but incredibly important thing we provide is a bed to lie in. This for me is a symbol of being attended to. We have gotten so inured to thinking that we can put any patient in a chair. And I think it's just gone too far."

Still, even now, in a waiting room teeming with patients and a staff stressed beyond belief, there are glimmers of humanity. Larry may have spent hours sitting in a chair, but a harried triage nurse found just enough time to get the blood work he needed before his CT scan, an IV to keep him hydrated and a dose of painkiller to ease his discomfort.

I look on FirstNet for the next patient. Cynthia turns her attention to a stack of orders for patients and starts printing labels for blood work.

"Thanks for looking after Larry," I whisper to her.

"We do what we can," she replies. The look on her face says it's killing her that she can't do more.

CHAPTER THREE

UNATTACHED

9:00 p.m.

"Brian, can I talk to you about a patient?" Ahu has a certain quality that marks her as a budding leader of the tribe of ER physicians. She has equipoise, which I define as the balance between wonderment and world-weariness.

"Are we frustrated?" I ask rhetorically.

"Yes," she sighs. "My patient is a twenty-eight-year-old guy named Bill who has pain in his left buttock and testicle. It started seven months ago and shows no sign of letting up. Have you seen him?"

"No, I haven't," I reply. "Why do you ask?"

"Because just about everyone who works here has." She launches into a recitation of the lengthy array of tests that Bill has had since his first visit to the ER: An ultrasound of his scrotum to make sure his testicle wasn't twisted and in danger of dying from lack of blood flow and oxygen. A CT scan of his abdomen and pelvis to check for a cancer lurking deep inside his body. An MRI of his spine to see if his pain is caused by a faulty sensory nerve to his butt. Blood tests to see if his sacroiliac joint—the joint that links the pelvis to the lower spine—is inflamed. Urine tests to see if he has an infection. Every one of those tests has come back normal.

Ahu then lists off the impressive array of specialists Bill has seen. These include a urologist, a rheumatologist and a neurologist. None of them could find anything wrong with him.

Each of those tests and specialist appointments has been arranged by an ER physician.

"I think it's time I meet him," I tell Ahu.

Even before I lay eyes on Bill, I'm starting to think about what might ail him. There are two kinds of pain. The most common is called nociceptive pain, which is pain caused by a diseased or broken body part. Think tumour, an inflamed appendix or a severely arthritic joint. Most of the tests and scans that doctors have at their disposal are good at diagnosing the sources of nociceptive pain. Because Bill's tests have all been negative, it suggests strongly that he does not have nociceptive pain.

The other kind of pain is known as neuropathic pain. This is pain that is generated by damaged or diseased nerves. Common causes include shingles and nerve damage resulting from diabetes. Could this be the culprit?

I follow closely as Ahu leads her patient to a stretcher in a cubicle that's kept empty for quick assessments a few feet from where I saw Larry. Bill appears young and fit but walks with a bit of a limp, as though he's favouring his left hindquarter. He winces when his left buttock lands on the stretcher a bit harder than he expected.

"Stretchers aren't built for comfort," I tell him. I offer my elbow, which Bill promptly bumps. "I'm Dr. Goldman. Ahu has told me about your pain and what my colleagues have done to try to sort it out. Why did you come to the ER tonight?"

There are two cardinal questions that ER physicians always ask. Both begin with the word *why*: Why have you come to the ER? And, Why now?

"The pain is not going away," says Bill with obvious frustration. "It used to come and go, but lately it's there almost all the time, especially at night. It's affecting my sleep."

This observation pricks up my ears. My clinical mentors taught me that sleep disruption can be a symptom of a potentially serious disease.

"Does the pain wake you from sleep?" I ask.

"Not so far," says Bill. "I've just noticed that the pain is there as I try to fall asleep. It's like I'm having trouble getting comfortable enough to sleep."

"It's reassuring that the pain isn't waking you up," I tell him. "That plus the fact that your tests and scans over the past few months have come back normal suggest that you don't have a serious medical condition. I suspect you have pain caused by nerve damage. The good news is that there are lots of possible treatments that work."

Ahu checks her notes. "The last ER doctor who saw Bill referred him to the chronic pain clinic. He's still waiting for an appointment."

"Unfortunately, that's not surprising," I say to Bill. There aren't nearly enough pain specialists and pain clinics to meet the needs of all patients. Wait times for appointments are often measured in many months, if not years. "Your family doctor should be able to prescribe some treatments that can help with this kind of pain."

"I don't have a family doctor," he says.

"May I ask why not?"

"He retired a couple of years ago," Bill says. "I haven't been able to get a new one."

"Okay. For now, I can start you on a medication that treats the kind of pain I think you have," I tell him. "The first pill may not work at the starting dose, or it may need to be increased or switched for a different medication. You really must find a family doctor who can make those kinds of adjustments for you."

"What if I can't?" Bill asks.

I hand the prescription to him. "Then come back to the ER if your pain gets worse." This is what we advise every patient we see in the ER.

As Ahu and I walk out of the cubicle and into the hallway, I can see she's still frustrated.

"He's been coming here for seven months," she says. "It's like we've become Bill's family doctor."

"How would you feel if you had a mystery pain like Bill's and didn't have a family doctor to turn to?"

When I started working in the ER back in 1982, emergency physicians saw family doctors as partners in a kind of relay race. Patients were the proverbial baton we passed back and forth. Family doctors took care of their patients thoroughly until illness or injury demanded emergency care. We handled the emergency (plus or minus a hospital admission) and sent the patients back to their family doctors when the crisis had passed.

More and more these days, our relay partner is unavailable or absent. On this shift alone, Bill is the fifth patient I've seen who doesn't have a family doctor, and I'm only two hours in. Experts call these people "unattached" or "orphan" patients. They not only put pressure on the hospital system but also tend to suffer worse outcomes and often don't get a diagnosis until their conditions are much more advanced and harder to treat.

Over sixteen months in 2022 and 2023, the OurCare research group surveyed 10,000 Canadians about their experiences with primary care and then collected the results in a report that was published in February 2024. Dr. Tara Kiran, a family doctor at St. Michael's Hospital in Toronto and OurCare's principal investigator, said, "I think it's one of the largest, most comprehensive surveys on not just people's experience with primary care, but also their values, their preferences, what they'd like to see in a future, better primary care system."

Among other things, the report revealed that 6.5 million Canadians, or more than one in five, don't have access to a family physician or nurse practitioner. Over 30 per cent of people in Quebec and Atlantic Canada lack primary care, and younger Canadians are the least likely to have a family doctor.

"Primary care is falling short," Kiran told CBC News when the survey results were published. "Far too many people don't have access to what is the front door to the health-care system. We're a country of have and have-nots. So many people have absolutely nothing—no access—and I think that's shameful, actually."

The impact on ERs of diminished access to primary care is enormous. In 2022–23, there were 15.1 million visits to ERs across Canada, according to the Canadian Institute for Health Information (CIHI). That was up from 14 million in 2021–22, a nearly 8 per cent increase in ER visits at a time when the annual population increase was hovering around one per cent. Some of those visits were undoubtedly triggered by Covid, but not all of them.

The number of unattached patients varies by province, but frontline workers right across Canada say it's a major factor in the current ER crisis as they experience it. "We have 30,000 unattached patients and people will say, 'Oh, that's not many compared to other provinces,'" said Dr. Trevor Jain, an emergency physician at the Queen Elizabeth Hospital in Charlottetown, PEI. "But we're a province of 165,000. So 30,000 is significant for us." (In fact, it's 18 per cent of the province's population.)

Jain told me that the system as currently designed does not work when you take family doctors out of the mix. He compares it to a football team without a quarterback. And when you add the growing numbers of patients with increasingly complex diseases and treatment regimens, it's a recipe for disaster. "You have

Canadians with chronic illnesses that are orphaned," said Jain. "The emergency department has become everything to everybody all the time."

When Don McLennan and Leah deForest moved to Nova Scotia from Manitoba in 2021, they joined an estimated 160,000 other residents on a very long wait list to get a family doctor. (That's 16 per cent of Nova Scotia's population of around 1 million people.) This came as a shock because the couple had easy access to primary care in Winnipeg. "We lived a five-minute walk from our doctor's place, and we were able to get an appointment definitely within a week," said Leah when I met with her and Don at their tidy little place in Martins Brook, a picturesque waterfront village ninety kilometres west of Halifax and a stone's throw from Lunenberg.

Don told me that if you need in-person care and you don't have a family doctor, your options are few. There are two walk-in clinics close to Martins Brook, but they have limited space and competition is heavy for coveted appointments. When the phone lines open at 8:30 a.m., you call like mad. "It's just the luck of the draw if your call goes through," he said. "I was never successful. If your call doesn't go through, you can be pretty sure that it's booked up for the day by 8:35."

Having come from a place where she had a doctor and hands-on care, Leah said she has found this very disturbing. "I don't want to go to emergency unless it's really an emergency. I don't want to clog that up. We've heard stories of people going to renew their prescriptions in emergency—and, I mean, that is not what you want to be doing."

Even in the bustling city of Halifax, things aren't much better. At some point or another, most unattached patients end up in overcrowded ERs. "There's such a lack of family physicians in Halifax and we have a growing population," said Dawn Gavin, a veteran triage nurse at Queen Elizabeth II Health Sciences Centre. Walk-in clinics are the next best option, but despite their name, she said, you can't just walk in and expect to be seen. "You have to make an appointment to be seen at those clinics," she explained. And all too often, as Don and Leah discovered, appointments are hard to come by.

Like other provinces, Nova Scotia does operate an 811 service that provides access to registered nurses who give non-emergency health information and advice. That almost certainly keeps some people from visiting the ER when they don't need to, but it's not a cure-all. "They follow a flip chart," Gavin told me. "The last page of the flip chart says to go to the emergency department, whether it's right away, in twelve hours or twenty-four hours. But it all comes back down to the emergency department."

At 14.78 per cent of the population, Ontario has one of the lower rates of unattached patients in Canada. Still, ER physicians in that province say people who lack primary care are placing emergency departments under unprecedented stress. Dr. Steve Flindall told me that orphan patients add to both the volume and the complexity of the patients they see at the suburban ER where he works.

"We're seeing lots of patients who don't have a family doctor," said Flindall. "I'm not saying that they've come to the emergency department *because* they don't have a family doc—they've come because they have an advanced state of illness. It's not that it hasn't been well managed. It hasn't been managed at all."

Even those who have a family doctor may not be able to get timely access to appointments. Flindall and his colleagues see plenty of patients like that. "People who have been slipping into congestive heart failure for months and haven't been able to get in to see their family doctor," he said. "As soon as you lay eyes on this person, you do a quick exam, you know they've got heart failure.

We've seen a lot of that." By the time these patients come to the ER, their illnesses are both life-threatening and harder to treat.

Dr. Paul Parks, of Medicine Hat Regional Hospital, noted that emergency physicians in his province are increasingly doing the work of family doctors. "We are actually diagnosing and treating hypertension in the emergency department," he said. In the ER, they start patients on blood pressure pills and bring them back in a week or two to see how they're doing. "That's just not how the system should function," he says. "There is just no other option."

And it's not just high blood pressure. These days, ERs are seeing lots of patients with unmanaged type 2 diabetes who have diabetes-related kidney failure and require dialysis. Patients with poor circulation who have infections that have gone into the bones of their feet. Patients with untreated osteoporosis who have nerve and spinal cord damage caused by collapsed vertebrae. With good primary care, much of that could be staved off, if not prevented altogether.

When the impact on the ER of this lack of primary care is tallied, one disease stands above the rest, and that's cancer. Some of the sickest and most tragic orphan patients have undiagnosed cancer. Almost every ER physician I interviewed for this book had at least one story. Some have many.

On a recent shift, for example, Paul Parks saw a sixty-two-year-old patient with increased respiratory distress. He ordered a CT scan and soon diagnosed metastatic lung cancer. "These are the diagnoses that we're making in the emergency department. That's on top of your regular traumas, respiratory infections. The pathology and the complexity of the stuff we're seeing now is crazy."

What's even stranger is that this patient was one of two that Parks diagnosed with metastatic cancer on the same shift. "I saw a thirty-four-year-old man who I diagnosed with stage four brain cancer," he recalled. "He had warning symptoms for a long time: clumsiness, trouble finding words, and headaches." Parks ordered a CT scan of the man's brain and saw a large tumour. Brain cancers are either primary, which means they originate in the brain, or secondary, which means they have metastasized to the brain from another part of the body, such as the lungs. Parks says the tumour looked like a metastasis. "You do a quick lookup at the patient's chart and it's metastatic, and it's quite obvious this patient's had symptoms for a long time," he said. "If they had a GP, I'm certain things could have got picked up sooner."

The cancers vary, but the scenario is often quite typical: an unattached patient arrives in the ER with ominous symptoms, such as a headache that isn't relieved with acetaminophen, or abdominal pain and jaundice. The ER physician orders a CT scan or ultrasound and it shows a mass that most likely is an undiagnosed cancer.

"I've diagnosed more cancer in the last three or four years than in my previous twenty," said Flindall. "I am seeing lots of people diagnosed with stage four pancreatic cancer [and] breast cancer who didn't have regular mammograms. They didn't get regular mammograms [because] there was nobody to prompt them to get tested."

Dr. Amy Nason, of the QEII Health Sciences Centre, told me she diagnoses a new cancer at least once every second or third shift. "We definitely see a lot of later presentation cancers because a lot of the screening stuff hasn't been happening or people aren't accessing it," she said. "Not only is this cancer but this is 'big deal' cancer. We can try and send you for treatment, but I expect that there will be nothing that will be curative, because we're picking it up late in the game."

It's distressing for ER physicians like Nason to tell patients they have advanced cancer. But that's nothing compared with what it's like to be on the receiving end of the diagnosis. "It's got to be horrible for people to meet someone like me for the first time ever and have me say, 'Hi, I'm spending five minutes with you. And then I'm going to come back in two hours after your CT scan and I'm going to change the course of your life forever. And then you'll never see me again.'"

Dr. Al Drummond, an ER and family physician in Perth, Ontario, and former medical director of the Perth and Smiths Falls District Hospital, paints a grim and emotional picture of what it's like to diagnose cancer in the ER.

"I've been moved to tears on some occasions seeing people with delayed diagnoses of cancer," he told me. "I think how bizarre and perverse [it is] that you show up in the emergency department and I'm telling you that you're going to die within the next three months and I just met you ten minutes ago. I'm wearing a mask and we're in a not very private space."

Social media has become a repository for stories about people's health and their experiences with the healthcare system. Kim Gaetz knows what it's like to be on the receiving end of a cancer diagnosis in the ER. On X she goes by the handle @kim_gaetz. In August 2024, she posted about being told in an ER that she had cancer of the ovary, and wondered if having a family doctor might have meant an earlier diagnosis.

"I am now seven months out since my ER diagnosis and still recovering," Gaetz told me in an interview. "The support from X was what got me through all the wondering and waiting and dark thoughts. The messages I got were overwhelmingly positive. I wish I had a family doctor throughout this process instead of going it alone."

So do I.

ER physicians aren't just telling patients they have cancer and bearing witness to their tears. Increasingly, they're fretting about the next step and trying to at least steer them in the right direction. For unattached patients, there is no quarterback to do what's needed to get the cancer staged and start the patient's treatment. In Charlottetown, Dr. Trevor Jain agonizes over what comes next. "I think the honest answer is we don't know what to do with them."

Dr. Keerat Grewal is trying to figure that out. She's a young physician in Toronto who, in 2024, was awarded a three-year Canadian Institutes of Health Research (CIHR) project grant to lead a multidisciplinary mixed-methods study examining the care of patients in Ontario who are diagnosed with cancer in the ER. She and her colleagues found that one in three people recently diagnosed with cancer visited an ER in the ninety days before a biopsy-proven diagnosis. "It's a huge number," said Grewal. "We can't say for certain if the diagnosis was made in the emergency department, but with that relatively short window, we think that [the visits are] probably related to the cancer diagnosis."

Just how many of those patients are unattached is unknown, but the very notion that one in three of them went to an ER in the three months prior to diagnosis suggests significant gaps in primary care. Grewal told me three likely scenarios are driving patients to the ER. "They don't have a family doctor, they can't access their family doctor for a couple of weeks or months down the line, or the family doctor has ordered imaging and it's not getting done in a timely way. So they're either sent to the emergency department or they come to the emergency department on their own to try and expedite that imaging."

Grewal is especially interested in studying the current system of cancer diagnosis and staging that Trevor Jain finds so frustrating—that murky pathway from abnormal CT in the ER to an appointment with an oncologist.

"To be seen by an oncologist, you'll need that tissue diagnosis to confirm malignancy," she said. "Overwhelmingly, most hospitals require that tissue diagnosis." This means that instead of referring a patient to an oncologist, the ER physician must first find a specialist who does biopsies and follows up on the results.

Jain tries to inch the patient down that road as much as he can. "I'll order a CT biopsy," he said, referring to a procedure that uses a CT scan to locate abnormal tissue and help pinpoint the place to get the biopsy. "But now you're locked into following the pathology," he said, meaning he feels an obligation to follow the patient's results until a tissue diagnosis is made. And yet, as he put it, "I'm not a cancer guy. I'm not a cancer doctor." Jain also told me that when he does eventually call in the "cancer guy," he may get a less than helpful response. Consultants can sometimes be "obstructive," he says, due to their own pressures, barriers and waiting lists.

I don't think a specialist has ever refused my request to see a patient who likely has cancer. But what I have experienced are bureaucratic rules that make it difficult, if not impossible, for the patients we see in the ER to get the cancer diagnosis and treatment they need.

"There's often not a straightforward path to get them to an oncologist," agreed Grewal. "We often send a referral for further workup, but we don't know whether patients make it to that follow-up. Oftentimes these referrals get lost or rejected."

Years ago, I figured out that the best way to avoid that is to refer the patient to be admitted to the hospital even when it isn't medically necessary. One of the most maddening things about the current system of cancer referrals out of the ER is that some hospitals grasp the problem, and some do not. Some throw up barriers, while others recognize that failing to deal expeditiously with cancer diagnoses leads to costlier downstream effects. To avoid that, the hospitals that get the problem encourage faster referrals to an oncologist, who arranges the biopsy and gets the patient into appropriate cancer care.

Keep in mind that these necessary logistical steps take place in the chaotic environment of the ER. Like every other doctor, Grewal has had those initial conversations with patients she's just met in hallways and in waiting rooms.

Grewal hopes her research will raise awareness of the scale and challenges of diagnosing cancer this way. "Hopefully this CIHR grant will show that this is a system-wide issue," she said. "And then we can turn our heads to how can we improve the system for patients."

Grewal doesn't believe that ERs should be the go-to place for patients who need a cancer diagnosis. "We should be adequately supporting our ambulatory care colleagues in order to keep these patients out of the emergency department," she told me. "But right now, with all the system-level issues that we're having, it's going to continue to be an issue. If you can't get a CT scan through the ambulatory care route and the only way you can get a same-day or next-day CT is through the emergency department, patients are going to come."

Grewal is now researching the effect that having to deliver this awful diagnosis has on the morale of her colleagues. "Emergency physicians feel frustrated that they can't care for these patients properly," she told me. "I feel like there's a lot of . . . emergency physicians [who] don't feel supported trying to get their patients to a cancer diagnosis and ultimately to an oncologist, and that we need more resources to be able to appropriately manage these patients" on an outpatient basis.

There's no question that the current situation is awful for patients and frontline providers alike, and Dr. Steve Flindall wonders whether justice has departed healthcare.

"It's like the system is privileging people who have good access to primary care over people who don't," he said. "If it's a publicly funded system, then all patients are equal. They should all have equal access to cancer screening and chronic disease management and counselling and all the things that, without which, they're going to end up [in the emergency department] in an advanced state of unwellness."

That as many as 6.5 million Canadians don't have access to primary care means there aren't enough family doctors and nurse practitioners to go around. This state of affairs did not happen overnight.

The arithmetic of primary care coverage in Canada is daunting, but there's no question we lag behind other Organisation for Economic Co-operation and Development nations. To merely reach the OECD average, Canada must increase the supply of family doctors over and above any increase in population growth. A close look at the numbers suggests we're not doing that. Between 2021 and 2023, the increase in the number of family physicians was just one per cent, while population growth ranged from 0.6 per cent to 2.9 per cent. And that doesn't account for all the family physicians who retire, quit, move away or die.

In 2022, *The Globe and Mail* analyzed statistics from the Canadian Institute for Health Information, or CIHI. The main headline from the data was that close to one in six Canadian family doctors are age sixty-five and older. The *Globe* reported that these doctors "make up the fastest-growing share of family doctors, with the percentage 65 and older more than doubling to 15 per cent from 6.5 per cent over the past 20 years." At the same time, there's been a corresponding drop in the percentage of doctors ages forty to forty-nine.

Reaching the age of retirement does not necessarily mean family doctors retire. For physicians, the concept of retirement is fuzzy and often not a binary choice between having a full practice and being out of medicine entirely. There are the doctors who would like to retire but feel obligated to carry on. In 2024, CTV's Avis Favaro reported that Dr. Peter Petrosoniak, a family doctor in Lindsay, Ontario, was still practising at age seventy-three. He said that he had planned to retire at seventy-two "but put it off because he [wasn't] able to find any physicians willing to take over his practice" of 1,400 patients plus 400 others he sees "on an ad hoc basis." The happy update to this story is that Dr. Sarah Ebhomien, a young family doctor, took over his practice in September 2024.

Petrosoniak's patient load may sound like a lot, but on average, family doctors are seeing fewer patients than they once did. In 2024, the CIHI reported that "the average number of patients seen by a family physician per year has decreased, from 1,746 in 2013 to 1,353 in 2021." It's easy to attribute this trend to an understandable desire for better work-life balance, but I suspect that many family doctors are seeing fewer patients largely because the patients they have are more complex to manage.

Complexity is a hot topic in medicine. The term refers to patients with multiple chronic physical, emotional and cognitive conditions. They are incredibly time-consuming for family doctors to see in general practice and for ER physicians to see in the emergency department. They require extensive care, multiple providers and potentially frequent hospitalizations.

Older patients with complex illness are less prepared than younger patients to manage their own illnesses. That increases the burden on family doctors to arrange for care. Newcomers to Canada may arrive with severe, untreated illnesses. Compounding the challenge of unravelling those illnesses is the fact that many recent arrivals to Canada do not speak either of Canada's official languages.

Complexity and other factors contribute to a rapidly shrinking supply of family doctors at a time when Canada needs many more of them. So what are the prospects for replenishing that supply?

A quick check of medical school graduates isn't encouraging. In the past few years, there has been a precipitous decline in the number of med students who want to be family doctors. In 2015, 38 per cent of those applying for residencies in Canada ranked family medicine as their first choice, according to the Canadian Resident Matching Service, or CaRMS. By 2023, it was down to 30 per cent. Fewer medical students are choosing family medicine because they've heard the complaints family doctors have regarding office practice and want no part of it.

After the first of two annual residency matches in 2024, 268 spots in family medicine residency programs remained vacant. CaRMS says that's the highest number of unfilled family medicine spots since the match began in 1969. Alberta alone had forty-two vacancies. That sounds bad, but as John Gallinger, CEO of CaRMS, told the *Ottawa Citizen*, there were more family medicine residencies available than in the past—"In part," he said, "in response to the shortage of family doctors."

That increase in residency positions hasn't stopped leading voices in the field from speculating on why medical school graduates may not be interested in becoming family doctors. "This kind of reinforces what we have known in terms of the perception of family medicine as a viable career going down among medical students," Ontario Medical Association president Dr. Andrew Park told the *Ottawa Citizen*.

Med students see family medicine as a less-than-viable career option because that's what practising family doctors have been telling them for years. They are dissatisfied with chronic issues. At the top of the list is relatively low pay. According to the CIHI, in 2020, family doctors grossed $287,000, while on average medical specialists earned $370,000 and surgical specialists earned $487,000.

And that's before overhead. The College of Family Physicians of Canada says that, compared with other specialists, family doctors on average spend a greater proportion of their gross income on overhead expenses, including such things as staff salaries, equipment leases, medical supplies and rent. For instance, across Canada in 2017, overhead expenses for family doctors averaged 28 per cent of gross income and 22 per cent for other specialties. In the ensuing years, the gap has widened.

To that, add unpaid paperwork. Family doctors typically spend ten to twenty hours a week on it without financial compensation.

If you're thinking that family doctors are greedy, I met a dedicated one recently who, after overhead, takes home around $60,000 a year. Would you be willing to settle for that given all the work and responsibility that goes with being a family doctor?

Moreover, family doctors feel disrespected by other specialists and by the public. And many—even younger ones in the prime of their careers—have been vocal about that.

Salt Spring is the largest of the Gulf Islands in the Georgia Strait between Vancouver Island and mainland British Columbia. In the summer of 2022, I arrived by floatplane, which is a bit of a luxury. The ferry is the usual way residents get to and from the island. That remoteness is what draws many people to Salt Spring, but it's also part of what makes it challenging to practise family medicine there, as Dr. Chris Applewhaite has discovered.

Applewhaite is an athletic, muscular man in his forties who does Brazilian jiu-jitsu and loves sea kayaking and fly-fishing. He was a physical therapist before going to med school at the University of Calgary. After he got his MD, he completed a residency in family medicine in Victoria and then spent two years in various places filling in for doctors on vacation and longer leaves.

In 2019, he arrived on Salt Spring Island with his wife, Aisia, and their daughters, Iris and Macy. The family chose Salt Spring because Aisia grew up on nearby Hornby Island and they saw it as a wondrous place to raise their kids. Applewhaite also saw it as a place where he could do the full scope of rural family medicine. Salt Spring is the only Gulf Island big enough to have its own hospital, and Chris was attracted by the opportunity to do regular turns in the ER and take care of inpatients as a hospitalist.

Just three years into his career, though, Applewhaite was thinking of quitting.

"I'll be honest, I think about it on a pretty regular basis," he told me back then. "The only reason that I'm doing it, and I think that most of us are doing it . . . right now, in this environment, is because we really care about our patients."

He showed me around the Salt Spring Island Health Centre, where he practised with five colleagues. He said two doctors were on their way out and only one was being replaced. The group, he said, had also struggled to maintain a full complement of administrative staff—it needs four office assistants to function smoothly but when I visited it only had two. The relatively low pay makes it difficult to hang on to employees.

He led me to a rectangular room with lots of computer workstations. He called it "the swamp." "This is the room where the paperwork happens, and family physicians everywhere have a significant amount of paperwork to do," he noted, referring to charts, requisitions for tests, notes to employers, insurance forms and more. "The burden of that has been increasing even in the time that I've been practising, which isn't that long."

The complaint about paperwork is universal among family physicians. I've spoken to many doctors who say they work a full day at the clinic and then, after a quick bite with the family and story time with the kids, spend their evenings filling out charts and forms. This is unpaid time. In BC, like other provinces, family doctors were paid only for patient visits. In 2022, the standard visit fee in BC was $33, comparable to the fee in most provinces.

Until recently, BC's fee-for-service system didn't compensate family doctors for taking on patients with more complex medical and mental health needs. Applewhaite told me about one patient who disclosed a history of trauma to him. The visit took much longer than the ten minutes he generally allocates to each patient so he can avoid creating a backlog in the waiting room. "I was not about to tell that patient, 'Listen, your ten minutes are up. It's time to go,'" he said. "I actually cancelled a few of my appointments that day, rescheduled them, so that she could have the time. At the end of the day, I'm getting $30 for the hour I spent with that patient."

Applewhaite had a gruelling schedule. He had a practice of a thousand patients at the clinic, where he worked three days a week. (He estimated that nearly half of the island's inhabitants do not have a family doctor. He's probably not far off. The CIHI reports that the number of unattached patients in rural and remote parts of BC is much greater than the national average.) Then there was his work at the Lady Minto Hospital, where he did seven to ten twelve-hour shifts in the ER each month. He also worked one out of every six weeks as a hospitalist, taking care of up to ten admitted patients. On those weeks, he was also second on call to the ER; he got called in when wait times were more than six hours and there were patients who required complex care.

When I spoke with him, what bothered Applewhaite more than the gruelling hours and low pay were the high rates of "moral injury" he said he and his colleagues were experiencing because of the limitations on their ability to provide care and the impact of that on patients. (Moral injury is widely understood to be the strong cognitive and emotional response triggered by circumstances and events that violate a person's moral or ethical code.)

He told me about recently diagnosing a patient with a brain tumour. "I consulted a neurosurgeon who suggested that the patient should get an urgent MRI of the brain to fully describe what was going on, and so she could have a real conversation about the prognosis and diagnosis with a neurosurgeon and/or oncologist," he said. The patient was told that the MRI was going to take three to four weeks to obtain. Meanwhile, her condition was deteriorating rapidly. In the end, she decided to have medical assistance in dying rather than wait for the MRI and risk suffering in the meantime.

"Of course, many people choose medical assistance in dying," Applewhaite continued, "but I think every patient deserves to have the full set of information in front of them before they decide to go that route. And more and more, that's not happening. People are just sort of throwing their hands up going, 'I know it's bad and I don't know when I'll get to see the cancer doctors, so I'm going to go this route.'"

BC is unique in that it is arguably doing more than most other provinces to address the root causes of despair and frustration among family doctors. In October 2022, the province announced a new payment model for family physicians. The model replaced the old fee-for-service system with one that paid physicians more to manage complex patients. It's called the longitudinal family physician, or LFP, payment model, and the fees it pays are calculated based on patient volume and complexity. For doctors like Applewhaite, this meant better compensation to help patients who are dealing with severe emotional or mental health challenges and seniors with health issues such as heart and lung conditions, kidney failure or dementia.

Under the new model, family doctors also finally started to be paid for time spent performing non-clinical duties like paperwork and reviewing X-ray and lab results. According to the province, the new framework would pay the average family physician an eye-popping gross annual income of $385,000, up from an average of $250,000 under the fee-for-service system.

The BC program went into effect on February 1, 2023. By the

end of 2024, over 4,000 of the province's 5,000 family doctors had signed on. Applewhaite was one of them. He told me that the changes have provided a financial lift. "Working in a clinic now feels financially sustainable," he said, and he has greater flexibility in how much time he can spend with his patients. But to him, the single greatest improvement is getting some compensation for previously unpaid work. "I have to admit there was a palpable sense of jubilation and validation that the huge amount of non-clinical work we are expected to do was finally being acknowledged."

The program has earned high-fives from BC family doctors like Robin Craven, who practises in Oliver, near the south end of the Okanagan Valley. "I think [with] what the B.C. government has done . . . we are attracting physicians from other provinces," she told CBC News in February 2024. Dr. Renee Fernandez, executive director of BC Family Doctors, the political voice of family doctors in the province, concurred. "What we're actually seeing is family doctors are staying in the system and we're seeing new family doctors join family practice for the first time in a generation."

Most everyone agrees that this has been a huge step in the right direction. But for Applewhaite and other BC doctors who have signed on to the program, their joy at getting more pay is tempered by the burden of paperwork that continues to rise alongside the increasing complexity of modern healthcare, coupled with growing requirements by the province to demonstrate accountability for money spent on healthcare through onerous documentation. Applewhaite told me that overall job satisfaction in primary care remains low and the rate of attrition remains high. "We have not experienced an increase in MDs in our community as a result of the changes to remuneration," he said. "And in fact the number has continued to decline."

Applewhaite admitted that he still thinks about quitting his clinic to work full-time in the ER or an urgent care clinic or as a hospitalist. "For now I'm pressing on," he told me, "hoping that things will get better for patients and the dedicated family doctors trying to take care of them. For all the troubles, primary care does still bring moments of joy, deep satisfaction and continuous challenge. Many of these moments are directly a result of the long-term relationships we have with our patients."

9:15 p.m.

I catch Ahu and Bill talking in the hallway. Bill heads towards the exit clutching a small sheaf of papers. There's something different about him. His bearing is lighter. He's almost smiling.

"What did you do to turn around his mood?" I ask my resident.

"I offered to take him on at my family practice clinic," she says.

"That was good of you."

"No worries," she says. "I'll be able to gain some extra tips on managing chronic pain."

"Bill's fortunate to have you as his family doctor," I tell her.

As a family practice resident spending time in the emergency department, Ahu has that option to offer our patients. I've never been a family doctor. I used to feel pleased inside when ER patients asked if I could be their family physician. These days, not being able to do that fills me with sadness for them.

But not for Bill. At least not this night. One unattached patient down. Several million more to go.

CHAPTER FOUR

MARKING TIME

9:30 p.m.

"Brian, can I talk to you about a patient in AZ?" Linus approaches me with pleading eyes. "Tawny is swamped and asked me to ask you if you'd mind reviewing this patient."

AZ is short for ambulatory zone. That's where we put patients with minor issues like cuts, broken bones and eye complaints. As each new doctor arrives, the ones already on duty move to zones whose patients have less urgent complaints. After their turn in AZ, they stop seeing new patients altogether and spend the remainder of their shift wrapping things up. As the doctor on the casino shift, I'm not due to start seeing patients in the AZ for another three hours. Like I said, it's busy.

Linus is a physician assistant, or PA. Physician assistants aren't MDs but advanced practice clinicians who are trained at medical schools. (In early 2025, the College of Physicians and Surgeons of Ontario began granting licences for PAs.) They see patients under the direct supervision of a licensed physician like me. By contrast, nurse practitioners, or NPs, practice independently of MDs.

PAs and NPs have been called "physician extenders" because they increase the number of patients we're able to see and the number of services we can provide. They take medical histories, do physical exams, order and interpret lab tests and diagnostic imaging and prescribe medications. What else they do depends on the physician or surgeon who's supervising them. For instance, PAs who work alongside orthopedic surgeons can become quite adept in the operating room at opening and closing incisions for hip and knee replacements.

The first PAs in the United States were military medics who served during the Vietnam War and later found jobs in the civilian healthcare sector. In 1984, the Canadian Armed Forces began using PAs as senior medics. The first formally trained PAs in Canada came from the ranks of the military. Today, there are civilian PA education programs at McMaster University, the University of Manitoba, the University of Calgary and Dalhousie University. There's also a PA Consortium program that's delivered collaboratively by the University of Toronto, the Northern Ontario School of Medicine and the Michener Institute of Education at the University Health Network.

I've worked alongside Linus for seven years. Like my physician and nurse practitioner colleagues, Linus is a committed and compassionate medical professional who often stays well past the end of his shift. Though he's eligible to claim overtime, he never does.

"You know I can't refuse you, Linus," I tell him. "But what are you getting me into?"

"I've got this fifty-two-year-old woman who dropped a shot glass on her right foot," he says, leading me to a small waiting area in the ambulatory zone.

"Anabel, this is Dr. Goldman." Linus hands me her emergency chart and gets down on his knees to point at a small cut on the top of her foot. "She's pretty sure there's a piece of glass stuck inside."

"I'm really sorry," says Anabel. "I realize this isn't a true emergency, but my foot hurts. I tried a walk-in clinic, but they said they didn't have the proper equipment to remove it."

"It says here you came in at noon!" I blurt as I scan the top part of Anabel's chart.

"Has it been that long?" she asks. "I've lost track of time."

"We should be the ones apologizing," I reply.

"You and your colleagues have had far more important things to take care of than my foot."

"Well, let's see if we can make up for lost time," I say.

Linus leads Anabel and me to a room that's a bit more private. I note that she doesn't put weight on her injured foot.

"Why don't you hop up here?" Linus helps her onto a stretcher. There's a 3 millimetre open cut on the top of her foot.

"Do you feel like there's a piece of glass stuck in there?" I ask her as I don a pair of disposable gloves.

"I feel a sharp, pointy stab each time I plantar flex my toes," she says.

"You've got the technical language right," I tell her. "You must be a health professional."

"Close enough," she says. "My ex chaired the board of the hospital in a small town in northern Ontario."

Anabel is what we call an "insider." Our instinct is to see insiders as a threat because they know what we do and can tell exactly how and when we do things wrong. In my experience, there are two types of insiders—those who want and even demand special treatment, and those who see it as their moral duty to be treated like everyone else. So far, Anabel seems to fall into the second group, but I still feel wary and want to proceed with caution.

"I was wondering where your incredible patience comes from."

"Nearly every week, we had to deal with complaints from patients and their families about the wait."

I notice that she said "we." "Were you on the board as well?"

"Might as well have been," she says. "In a small town, everyone knows everyone else. Every person who wrote in to complain was someone I'd meet at the supermarket, the church or the one half-decent restaurant in town."

Looking closely at the cut, I can't see any glass poking out. With my gloved fingertip, I gently feel the cut and surrounding area on the top of Anabel's foot.

"Ouch!" she says. "You found it."

"Sorry about that," I tell her, taking a pen from a pocket and marking the spot with an *X*. "I'm sorry to make you wait longer, but I'd like to take an X-ray to see if we can locate the glass fragment more precisely. That way, when I freeze the top of your foot with local anesthetic, I'll know exactly where to look."

Linus and I walk over to a computer workstation. I look over his shoulder as he logs on to his account and orders an X-ray of Anabel's foot.

"Are you going to try to dig out the glass?" he asks.

"Try is the word," I reply.

My success rate at removing glass shards is fifty-fifty at best. I pray silently that I don't end up sending Anabel home after a twelve-hour wait with a sore foot and nothing to show for it.

ER insiders typically come from the ranks of frontline healthcare providers, but some, like Anabel, are healthcare adjacent—they don't directly provide patient care. And sometimes, an outsider can become an insider. I'm talking about someone who is an expert in a field outside of healthcare but has emotional skin in the game and powers of observation not compromised by illness or injury.

Someone like Joanne MacCormac, a woman I interviewed who has become something of an expert in what it's like for patients and loved ones to wait endlessly in the ER.

MacCormac is in her early sixties. She lives in Ottawa and has had a highly accomplished career in the complex world of the federal bureaucracy. At one point she was head of financial operations at the Department of Foreign Affairs. In her last post before retiring, she was the director at Indigenous Services Canada.

MacCormac is the mother of Shannon, a twenty-two-year-old with macrocephaly-capillary malformation, or M-CM, an ultra-rare genetic syndrome that causes overgrowth of the body and head along with abnormalities of the skin, blood vessels, brain and limbs. The disease is caused by mutations in a gene called PIK3CA. When the gene functions normally, it signals cells and tissues in the brain and the body to stop multiplying. The mutated gene fails to do that, so the cells and tissues under its command continue to grow and multiply without end. M-CM is so rare that it affects fewer than one in every million people.

MacCormac told me the effects on her daughter are profound. "It's impacted her balance and intellect," she said. "She's maybe functioning at a developmental age of one and a half to three years. She has limited verbal ability and was diagnosed with autism as well. She is incontinent. She is able to walk but not for long distances. She requires care twenty-four seven."

Currently, Shannon lives at home with MacCormac and her husband, John, a retired firefighter. Once Shannon aged out of the public school system, Joanne and John had to take on more of her care, which has been all-consuming, to say the least. Unless Shannon is placed in a long-term care home, their parental duties will also continue to grow and multiply.

But despite her limitations, Shannon is healthy, and MacCormac has had to rush her to the ER only on rare occasions. One of those happened recently, though, when Shannon's dad took her to an Ottawa recreation complex where they go every weekday to walk and get some exercise.

"This particular day," MacCormac explained, "John was walking about two or three metres behind Shannon and she just went down. She has a very high pain tolerance because of the developmental delay. John went to pick her up and she started to cry, which she rarely ever does. He knew something was wrong."

Shannon was unable to walk. Her dad summoned one of her sisters, and the two of them were able to get Shannon into a wheelchair the complex kept on-site. They got her into the car and drove her to the ER closest to their home. At 10:00 a.m., Shannon was registered to be seen. At 10:30, MacCormac arrived in the ER. She told me that a nurse assessed Shannon "maybe around 11:30." At that time, the nurse noticed some swelling and said, "She's definitely injured her ankle." At 11:45, the nurse gave Shannon acetaminophen. She doesn't swallow pills easily, so the nurse crushed the pain reliever and mixed it with applesauce.

"And then we waited," said MacCormac. "We sat and we waited in the waiting room."

Shannon sat in a wheelchair from 10:00 a.m. until 7:30 p.m. while her parents did what they could to keep their daughter comfortable. "We had her iPad," MacCormac recalled. "She doesn't wear headphones, so people around us could hear the iPad as well. We tried to give her some lunch, but she didn't want to eat—even her favourite treats, which was unusual for her."

Occupying the time of an adult daughter with profound developmental delay was not MacCormac's only concern. Because Shannon is incontinent, she wears adult diapers and needs to be changed regularly. She also has a pilonidal cyst, which is a fluid-filled sac under the skin at the top of the crease between her buttocks. Depending on how big the sac is, pilonidal cysts can be quite painful. They are also prone to infection.

MacCormac told me she asked the nurses to find a place in the ER where she could change her daughter. "They said we have no place," she recalled. "'We have no beds.'"

There was a public washroom nearby. Although MacCormac

could wheel Shannon to the washroom door, the injured ankle made it impossible for her to get Shannon safely inside the washroom and onto the floor where she could be changed. MacCormac asked one nurse if Shannon's foot could be placed in a boot so she could try to walk her daughter to the washroom. She was told that option wasn't possible until they'd determined whether Shannon had a fracture and how the fracture was to be managed.

At one point, mother and daughter found a relatively secluded spot in a waiting area directly in front of the X-ray room. But a staff member then said MacCormac had to wheel her daughter to a different waiting area around the corner.

"It was jam-packed," said MacCormac. "There was nowhere for us to find a spot where we were not in the way of staff and other patients."

Sometime around 7:30 p.m., Shannon was finally called in to have an X-ray taken of her foot. An hour later, a service assistant brought her back in because they needed another X-ray. "They did about four different X-rays on her foot and said there's a small fracture," MacCormac said.

Shannon was then seen by a resident in orthopedic surgery. Apparently, there was another abnormality on the X-ray that the resident could not identify on the X-rays that had been taken.

"'We'd like to get a CT scan of her foot,'" MacCormac recalled being told. The resident said it would take perhaps another forty-five minutes before the CT scan could be done.

By this point, another hour had gone by and Joanne still hadn't been given a place to change Shannon. She asked the orthopedic resident to advocate on her behalf. Finally, the nurses gave them a room where Mom could change her daughter. It was 8:30 p.m., some ten and a half hours after Shannon had been brought to the ER. The CT scan still hadn't been done. That was one wait too many.

"Shannon was done," MacCormac said. "I pulled all the tricks out of my hat to keep her as quiet and calm and happy as I could out in that waiting area, but it's exhausting."

Shannon was fitted with an Aircast, a prefabricated "controlled ankle motion" boot that's designed to bear weight while immobilizing or restricting movement of the foot, ankle and calf. The nurses told MacCormac that she'd be contacted by the hospital about a booking for the CT scan that hadn't been done plus a follow-up visit with the orthopedic surgeon on call. They finally left the ER at 9:00 p.m., eleven hours after Shannon was brought in.

"We didn't get discharge papers," MacCormac told me. "'Here's your Aircast. Here's how you put it on. You'll get a bill in the mail basically for the cast.' So that's kind of how we left the hospital."

MacCormac says she was not contacted for the CT scan or the appointment with the orthopedic surgeon. A week went by, and she finally called the surgeon's office herself and was told that her family doctor was supposed to order the CT scan. Her family doctor told MacCormac it was the job of the orthopedic surgeon.

"She went five weeks with no follow-up, no additional X-ray, no CT scan, no nothing," said MacCormac. "I think Shannon kind of fell between the cracks in terms of follow-up or additional care."

Shannon, the youngest of three daughters, has had special needs almost since birth.

First, she developed hydrocephalus, a condition in which too much fluid accumulates in the brain and the spinal cord. When she was six months of age, surgeons inserted a shunt in her brain to drain off excess fluid. Meanwhile, she was found to have poor balance and severe developmental delay. At eight and ten years of age, she required additional neurosurgical procedures to decompress her brain.

It was around the time of her third neurosurgery that Shannon was diagnosed with M-CM. "When Shannon was born, there were fewer than 300 cases in the world. Now it's maybe around 350, mostly in the United Kingdom and the United States," MacCormac said. "There's a couple of other cases in Canada now."

MacCormac was able to join a Facebook group of M-CM parents and gain support. "We parents were the ones that were leading any advancements in M-CM. Many of the doctors of those newborns had no idea what M-CM is."

MacCormac is also a member of "One More Thing," a Facebook group named sardonically for the endless list of demands faced by parents of kids with extraordinary medical needs. The group, based in Ottawa, is largely made up of mothers of children with complex diseases who meet to give advice and provide emotional support. They frequently compare notes on the encounters they have with frontline healthcare providers at clinics, in hospitals and in the ER.

The trip to the Ottawa ER was one of the first times Shannon had received care in an adult hospital since she aged out of the pediatric system. Based on considerable past experience with the healthcare system, MacCormac is certain that had she brought Shannon to a pediatric hospital, the triage nurse would have immediately identified her daughter as having special needs and Shannon would not have been left in the waiting room as she was in the ER intended mainly for adults. That assumes, of course, that there were no other children who required more urgent life-saving measures.

"It was our first experience in an adult ER, and unfortunately it was frustrating and long and disappointing," MacCormac told me. While they waited, she paid close attention to what was going on around her. Not surprisingly, she saw lots of people who were coughing and sneezing. She saw patients with foot injuries and a young man who was in the custody of two police officers. (He had his own room and stood in the doorway glaring at the rest of them.) "There was a woman in a wheelchair, and someone who was with her who held a plastic bag for her to vomit," she recalled. "She just couldn't keep anything down. I felt for her because she was obviously ill." Ill and left mainly to her own devices.

MacCormac said she wasn't the only patient or family member who was frustrated by the wait. "One of the men in the area where we were said he waited almost nine hours for a five-minute visit and a diagnosis which he already knew. He was quite perturbed as well."

At one point, she went to the triage station to ask when Shannon was going to get called for an X-ray. "I stood at that nurse's station door probably five, six, eight minutes and nobody noticed me," she said. "Finally, I tapped on the window. The nurse was as helpful as she could be. But I wouldn't say she was sympathetic, and I don't think any of them were what I would call compassionate."

While Shannon waited a long time, that wasn't the case for everyone. Joanne saw an infant around two years of age accompanied by a mother, and a grandfather who was brought in quickly and was in and out of the ER in two hours. "So maybe they triage younger children quicker than the others," she said.

Aside from that, she saw little if any evidence of special consideration for people with unusual needs. One elderly woman was suffering from severe back pain and another had fallen and broken her ankle quite badly. MacCormac overheard the doctor telling the second woman's family that she needed to be admitted for an operation. "She had waited just as long as Shannon had as well," she said. "So my observation is that they just don't have enough resources—meaning doctors, nurses and rooms. It's quite sad."

Is Shannon's story evidence that emergency medicine is on the verge of collapse, as some insiders have suggested? Perhaps a better word—the word that comes closest to what Joanne saw—is *overwhelmed*, starting with the physical space.

"The facility is not designed to hold that many people in that waiting area," MacCormac said of the ER where she took Shannon. "I mean, people are just spilling out. And it's just very sad to see that. You don't want to point the blame at the nurses who were there and who showed up for work. For that I give them credit. But the decency, the respect, down to the little gestures, were not there at all."

More than a month after the visit to the ER, and after MacCormac made multiple attempts to reach the orthopedic surgeon, Shannon finally got her follow-up appointment. The surgeon noted that the fracture was relatively small. He recommended that Joanne begin weaning Shannon off her Aircast.

Despite the injury and the eleven-hour ordeal in the ER, Joanne says Shannon has bounced back nicely. "She and John started back on the track with no hesitation," she told me. "She was more resilient than we thought she would be." I asked if she'd shared Shannon's experience with the "One More Thing" Facebook group, but she said she hadn't. "I haven't shared it because I don't know if it's that drastic compared to everyone's experience," she explained. "We've all kind of been there."

For Shannon and her mom, a relatively minor injury turned into an ordeal in the ER. It got me wondering what MacCormac will do when Shannon has a surgical emergency or a major illness like pneumonia or a kidney infection.

"Well, I would consider my options," she said. But what are those options? Joanne suggested that instead of a big-city ER, she could take her daughter to a smaller ER in a rural town like Arnprior, located some sixty-five kilometres west of downtown Ottawa. But as we'll find out, that could be a risky choice because ERs in rural towns are closing with alarming frequency.

"Maybe I would call an ambulance," she mused, "because at least she'd hopefully get a little bit faster attention." But as we've seen, given the increasingly lengthy offload delays that paramedics face when they bring patients to the ER, that would be unlikely to make Shannon's wait any shorter.

MacCormac is savvy enough to realize that there is no clear path for what she will do when the need arises. "It is going to happen someday [that] she will need that care," she said. "And will it be there?"

As bad as Shannon and her mom's uncomfortable wait in the ER was, it's nothing compared with what's experienced by patients who are waiting for a bed on an inpatient ward.

Take, for instance, Matthew Mukash, a seventy-three-year-old from Whapmagoostui, the northernmost Cree village in Quebec. Mukash also happens to be the former grand chief of the Cree nation of Eeyou Istchee, one of the most populous Indigenous nations in the province.

In January 2024, the former grand chief found himself reclining on a gurney crammed into a corner alcove in a hallway just steps from the entrance to the ER at Montreal General Hospital. The alcove had waist-high walls topped with glass, making it look more like a fishbowl than a private space for seeing patients. On the other side of the glass, a mirror-image alcove held another stretcher occupied by another patient. If you looked through the glass wall at the foot of Mukash's gurney, you would see stretchers on either side of a short hallway leading to the main doors.

He was in this hallway for four days.

Hundreds if not thousands of patients have languished in the hallways of Canadian ERs for days at a time just like Mukash. Their experiences are left to the imagination. His is not. That's because his son Pakesso recorded video of his dad for all to see.

"New people arriving regularly, some are even under the influence," Mukash says on the video, his son translating his Cree words into English. He wears a hospital gown with red-and-black pyjama bottoms. The fluorescent overhead lights bathe the hallway in an unending antiseptic glow. There's no night table. His only creature comfort appears to be a box of tissues. His grey hair is combed but his face looks weary. He clearly hasn't gotten much sleep during his hospital stay. "Some are aggressive and some have even wanted to fight. That's what I've seen."

For most of those four days and nights, Mukash's granddaughter Jade was at his bedside, or gurney-side. Jade is an artist and a youth representative at Cree Women of Eeyou Istchee Association. She has also worked at the Cree Board of Health and Social Services of James Bay. She says her grandfather had been having pain in his back for six months. "In January [2024] what we really saw that concerned us was a very large amount of weight loss, and that happened very quickly. So that was the reason to bring him to our local clinic in Whapmagoostui."

By that point, Mukash was so frail he needed a wheelchair. "I think even the doctors and nurses that saw him [at the clinic] were a little bit shocked, you know, to see that decline so quickly," Jade told me. "They were very quick to say that it was an emergency and that he needed to be sent to Montreal as the closest major centre."

Jade and her grandfather were transported by air charter from Whapmagoostui to Montreal with several stops along the way. It was a long and uncomfortable journey for Mukash. They arrived in the ER at Montreal General at 9:00 p.m. on January 7. A triage nurse assessed her grandfather, and because the ER wasn't too busy at the time, he was soon taken to an examining room. He had blood taken for testing and a CT scan of his spine. A few hours after arriving, Mukash was seen by an ER physician and then moved to another room inside the ER, where he and Jade spent the first night.

The ER doctor ordered additional scans but thought Mukash was well enough to be discharged, even though he was debilitated and in pain. "Sadly, I wasn't surprised," Jade said. "They often want to send us home right away." When she said that discharging him now would probably mean that the two of them would have to repeat the arduous trip in short order, the doctor reconsidered.

The next day, Mukash had the additional scans. A second ER doctor mentioned that he might have cancer and said he needed more tests. "It was a very big shock for us," said Jade. Her grandfather was then referred to the general internal medicine team on call to be admitted to the hospital. He was taken to the stretcher where he would spend the next four days. It was parked in the waiting room, directly across from the receptionists' workstation and steps from a security desk, with the aforementioned walls made of wood and glass. "We saw every single person that walked in to see reception," Jade recalled, "and a lot of people being wheeled by in their stretchers to go to their appointments or to go to their scans. It was right next to us." At night, the receptionists would talk loudly with each other to pass the time. "I think they weren't mindful that there were patients right in front of them," said Jade.

On top of the noise and lack of privacy, they had no call buttons, making it hard to get the attention of the nurses. "We had to get the receptionist to tell the nurse to come see us." The one time they did manage to speak to a nurse, her grandfather asked for a sleeping pill, but was told that a doctor was not going to provide one. "They were just overwhelmed," said Jade, "and there was nothing more that we could say or do to help the situation."

This went on for four days. Her grandfather did receive lots of blood tests, an MRI and a liver biopsy, but in between, Jade explained, it was hours and hours of sitting there with no updates. After they were told he might have cancer, nothing. "I don't think I heard the word 'cancer' again for the next four days," she said. "It was all kind of vague words like 'lesions' or 'lumps.' Nothing straight up."

Suddenly, it all came to an end.

"At the fourth day, they just told us, 'We're going let you go. You just have to go back home,'" Jade recalled. They were told that her grandfather would have follow-up appointments within a couple of weeks, but no one sat down with them and discussed the diagnosis and the plan for treatment.

"They just handed me papers," she said. She saw that her grandfather had been referred to the Cedars Cancer Centre, a major hub for cancer treatment and research in Montreal. "That's how we found out for sure what was going on. And I had to tell my grandfather."

The two left the hospital believing that Mukash, who was more debilitated than when he arrived, had an aggressive form of cancer and possibly only weeks to live. They spent a couple of days recuperating at the hotel where Jade had stayed while her grandfather was in hospital and then went home to Whapmagoostui. They weren't sure it was even worth returning to Montreal to begin treatment. But by the time he had his first appointment at Cedars a few weeks later, both the diagnosis and the prognosis had changed radically and for the better.

"It was actually a lymphoma," said Jade. "And even though the lymphoma was extremely aggressive, it's the kind that reacts well to chemo."

Instead of planning a funeral, Jade moved with her grandfather to an apartment in Montreal so that he could receive treatment. When I spoke to them, he had just completed his fifth round of chemotherapy. "He's doing great," she told me. "He's not in a wheelchair anymore. He's very independent. He's walking around a lot. Of course, the chemo is not easy, but I do see a big improvement in his health."

What Jade doesn't see is a big improvement in the ER anytime soon. In Whapmagoostui, she worked as a medical receptionist, so like Joanne and Anabel, she's an insider who understands how the system works and sees where it falls short. Her critique of what she observed in the ER at Montreal General is hard to hear but necessary. She told me that a few of the nurses looked tired and burnt-out. But most of them were a blur, moving so quickly from patient to patient that they scarcely left an impression.

"It was like there was no passion in the care," she said. "That's what I saw for a few of the people. The doctors we saw kept saying they're overworked or overtired and that they were doing the best they could."

Unfortunately, Indigenous people haven't always been able to count on getting the best care possible. Like other provinces, some hospitals in Quebec have treated patients like Mukash badly.

One patient treated exceptionally badly was Jade's mother, Natasia Mukash. In 2017, she testified about her experience at the Viens Commission, a two-year public inquiry headed by former Superior Court justice Jacques Viens. The commission started as an investigation into relations between Indigenous people and the Sûreté du Québec, the provincial police, after a news outlet published a story in which ten Indigenous women from the Val-d'Or region said they had been subject to abuse by officers. Over time, the commission's focus was broadened to include corrections, justice, youth protection and health and social services.

In May 2016, Natasia Mukash had a miscarriage followed by ten days of prolonged bleeding. She was transported by plane from Whapmagoostui to Val-d'Or, where she was taken to the hospital ER. While there, she overheard nurses talking in French, which they clearly assumed she couldn't understand. She heard one say, "She's from the north," followed by laughter. Mukash told the commission she was directed to a bathroom contaminated by vomit. Around midnight, about six hours after she'd arrived, a nurse told her she should leave in a taxi and stay at a hotel without seeing a doctor. But she refused to go. Eventually, she was taken to a room and hooked up to an IV. She testified that a nurse told her there had been a "misunderstanding." Mukash was so desperate for the mistreatment to end that she even apologized for refusing to leave the hospital.

At first, she blamed herself for the way she had been treated. She became depressed. "At one point, I questioned how I look, or my name. I didn't feel comfortable with myself," she testified before the commission. She said she eventually complained to the hospital but didn't receive a response.

Afterwards, the head of the commission thanked Mukash for her testimony. He also told her that she was right to sound the alarm about the way she was treated. "If you feel it was bad enough, I have the same feeling," Viens told her.

Jade said it was very difficult to see her mom testify and hear about all she had been put through. "Unfortunately," she told me, "it's something that a lot of other women go through."

Mukash's story was one of many heard by the commission. Some of those accounts were delivered not by patients but by frustrated healthcare providers. Dr. Samir Shaheen-Hussain, an ER pediatrician and professor at McGill University's Faculty of Medicine, told the commission that the treatment of Indigenous people is often so bad "that the patients brace themselves and devise strategies to 'decide how to deal with the racism . . . they will encounter when they walk into an emergency room.'"

The Viens Commission's final report, released in 2019, contained 142 recommendations, 34 of which addressed deficiencies in the provision of health services and social services. Those recommendations ranged from enshrining the concept of cultural safeguards, to working with Indigenous authorities in order to make emergency medical transportation services by land or air more readily available. Other recommendations addressed rehabilitation, addiction services, long-term care and end-of-life care.

The pace of improvement has been slow. In the first follow-up report, released in October 2023, only one of the thirty-four calls for action concerning health and social services had been implemented. Nine were reported to be "progressing as expected," and twenty-four "had not generated any satisfactory outcomes."

For patients and their loved ones, some waits are inconvenient. Some are painful. Some come with a lack of privacy and other indignities. But some have potentially serious medical consequences.

On a Sunday morning in late January 2024, Angelina Malott, a nursing student at Conestoga College in Kitchener, Ontario, got up at five feeling vaguely unwell. "I just thought I was tired or hungry," she explained. She tried eating, but that made her feel worse. She developed abdominal pain that grew more intense over the course of the day. "I was lying on the couch curled up and crying because I was in so much pain," she said.

Eventually she sought out Julia, the wife of Angelina's sister, Mandy. In their household, Julia is the one who fills the role of mother. "Yeah, I call her my kid," Julia told me. "She calls me her parent and she calls me her mom sometimes. I support this kid financially, emotionally and mentally. I care for this kid like my child."

Julia told me that Angelina is not a complainer by nature. "She knows her body well. By 8 or 9 p.m., she was crying about it and saying it just hurt so bad. And that's not normal for her to react that way."

Around ten that night, Angelina told Julia that she wanted to be taken to the hospital. Both of them knew that the wait at Kitchener ERs was likely to be long, but they grabbed their phones and a water bottle and headed off to St. Mary's General Hospital. "I just remember slowly walking up a slight hill and thinking, 'Oh my God, this is horrible,'" Angelina said.

She was triaged within ten minutes of her arrival. She remembers leaning against Julia and wanting to go home. Fifteen minutes later, she was taken inside the ER and given a bed. She felt cold and spent the next few hours dozing under warm blankets, waking up frequently because of pain or nausea.

"I'm thinking 1:45 to 2 a.m. was when we saw the doctor the first time," said Julia, noting that the wait for things to happen didn't seem outrageous to her. "Angelina had a bed she could lie down in, so at this point, this was going very much the way that I'm used to with our modern hospital system."

Around 4:00 a.m., the doctor came by and told them he thought Angelina had appendicitis. He said he was going to order an ultrasound to confirm the diagnosis, but since St. Mary's doesn't do ultrasounds at night, that meant she had to wait until the technician came in at 8:30 a.m.

In a situation like Angelina's, an ultrasound is essential to confirming the diagnosis. There are many other conditions that can look just like appendicitis, including gynecological issues like a ruptured ovarian cyst, twisting of the fallopian tubes around the blood vessels that nourish them or pelvic inflammatory disease, which is an infection of one or more female reproductive organs. Intestinal conditions such as Crohn's disease and infectious colitis can also mimic appendicitis. In my decades as an ER physician, I've seen all of these and others turn out to be the actual cause of right-sided abdominal pain, tenderness and nausea.

But at least for Angelina, the medications for pain and nausea had kicked in, and she began to feel a bit better. Then, at around five or six that morning, she was asked to vacate the stretcher and go back to the waiting room. "I don't think I was wearing my shoes," she told me. "I was just wearing socks." She got off the stretcher and pulled her IV along with her back to the waiting room. She remembers the IV kept beeping because the battery was low.

"This is where the experience started to go south for us," Julia said. "She lost her bed. They said they needed to give the bed to somebody else . . . So she is taken out of the bed and put back out into the waiting room and we're waiting till 8 a.m. I ask if we can take her home. We have beds at home. 'Can I take her there to let her sleep and I'll come back at 8 a.m.?' But of course we can't do that."

Angelina found herself sitting in a corner of the waiting room, close to an outlet to recharge her IV. There were empty chairs all around her. The waiting room wasn't full of people. Meanwhile, Julia went home to fetch a bag of clothes, toiletries and some books. At one point, a guy asked the nurse if he'd lose his place in the queue if he went to get food from the Tim Hortons inside the hospital. The nurse told him he could leave and come back, no problem. "The reason why I remember that is because he got an ultrasound before I did," said Angelina. "I was very, very frustrated with that."

When Julia got back to the ER, she could see that Angelina was not doing well. "She's sitting in one of those uncomfortable hospital chairs," she told me. "Every time she's in too much pain she starts to cry and makes sounds, and the nurse comes and puts more drugs in [her IV]."

Around 9:10 a.m., Angelina was finally called in for her ultrasound. At about ten, she found out that she needed to be transferred to Grand River Hospital. "A new doctor comes and tells us that they got the ultrasound done, [and] it *is* appendicitis," said Julia. "She will need surgery [but] they can't do the surgery here [at St. Mary's]. I've now learned that in Kitchener-Waterloo, appendicitis surgeries are always done at Grand River Hospital, so they always do a patient transfer when someone needs an appendectomy."

I asked Julia whether Angelina's appendix had burst. This detail was not clear at this point in her story. "I didn't know this yet," Julia explained, "but I would later find out when I got the report from the hospital that the ultrasound was conclusive that she had appendicitis—they could see the inflammation—but it was not conclusive whether or not she had a ruptured appendix."

A ruptured or burst appendix is a big deal. I've heard of patients who have died of complications following a ruptured appendix. Thirty-six hours after symptoms begin, the risk is roughly 2 per cent. After that, the risk jumps by another 5 per cent every twelve hours. At this point, Angelina had been experiencing pain for more than twenty-four hours.

A CT scan of the abdomen is considered the most accurate and sensitive imaging test for diagnosing appendicitis in adults. The main drawback is that it exposes the patient to radiation, which for young adults increases the risk of cancer later in life. Ultrasound does not involve such exposure, but it's less accurate and more likely to fail to visualize and identify an inflamed appendix. In those cases, if the doctor strongly suspects appendicitis, then a CT scan is usually done as a second test.

Because Angelina was a teenager, it was entirely appropriate for her to have an ultrasound first.

Assuming that the appendix can be seen, hypothetically speaking an experienced ultrasound radiologist can usually tell if the appendix has burst by identifying pus around the organ. In this case, Julia says there was some doubt. But Angelina's symptoms had been going on more than long enough for her to have a burst appendix. She needed exploratory surgery and an appendectomy.

With a diagnosis of a possibly burst appendix, you might think this would be the moment when the system kicks into high gear and gets things moving. But Julia said that didn't happen. The wait, now more than twelve hours and counting, groaned on. "I think I understood at that point that this was going to require some strong advocacy on our part," Julia told me. "And I know how to do that."

Much like Matthew Mukash's son, Julia turned to social media for help. "I have a tiny camera I keep in my purse . . . and I just had this feeling that . . . this might be a moment that some public awareness would be due." She started to take videos. A lot of them. And she posted them on X.

Julia produced a long thread describing Angelina's ordeal and aimed it at journalists and other prominent watchers of Canadian healthcare on social media. It took another day for Angelina's story to be covered by the CBC, CTV and other national media, but much sooner than that, she got action at the hospital.

"Pretty much exactly as I finished, the charge nurse came over to us and she had clearly been told about what was happening [the social media campaign] and had gotten some action on our situation," said Julia. The nurse gave her transfer documents to give to staff in the ER at Grand River, the name of the surgeon accepting Angelina for transfer and everything else needed to proceed.

Because no ambulance was available, Julia decided to drive Angelina to Grand River herself.

It was around 1:00 p.m. when they finally walked into the Grand

River ER. Angelina now had a proven diagnosis of appendicitis. Keep in mind that as time passes, the likelihood rises of a burst appendix and a much riskier and more complicated illness. But in the ER, Julia felt as if Angelina was treated like any patient who has just registered to be seen for the first time.

Julia says the staff at St. Mary's had written "day surgery" and the name of the surgeon on the front of the envelope containing the transfer papers that Julia brought to the ER. But she says that no one at Grand River had seen the transfer package because Julia says she wasn't able to catch anyone's attention to deliver it. In other words, it's possible that no one on duty in the ER that day knew that Angelina was coming with a confirmed diagnosis of appendicitis because they hadn't been informed.

As a veteran ER physician, my experience is that patients who are fully worked up at a referring hospital and have been accepted by a consulting service do not get back in line. Their care and disposition are generally expedited by the people who have accepted the patient. Instead, Julia says Angelina sat for another hour and a half. Her IV wasn't connected to fluids. She wasn't getting antibiotics to treat the possible infection in her belly. And she wasn't getting any painkillers.

"And this is where I lost it," Julia told me. "She has not been seen by triage. Nobody has talked to us since we came in there. No one has even come to see what we're there for."

Meanwhile, that long thread on X begins gaining traction. "My phone is dinging like nobody's business," Julia recalled, "because it is taking off at this point and getting hundreds of shares and retweets and comments as it gains attention."

That's when she decided to take things a step further. "I go back up to the nice elderly volunteer who checked us in and I start to have very strong words about what's happening with my daughter and the fact that nothing is being done."

The volunteer fetched the triage nurse, and from that point on, things changed. Angelina was immediately brought into triage, and the nurse was "very apologetic," Julia said. "I think then she understood the severity of this and the ridiculousness of it."

After her quick stop at triage, Angelina was immediately directed to day surgery because they were expecting her. She had a bed to get settled in. She was given pain medication. Two hours later, around 4:00 p.m., she was taken to the OR to have her appendix removed.

Meanwhile, Julia posted another video. "For the sake of Ontarians, I needed to capture this moment to try to change things and make things better," she explained.

Julia told me that she believes her interventions on Angelina's behalf worked even though they went against what she called a "quintessential Canadian desire to not impose." She believes Canadians don't like to complain about waiting because they don't want to be rude and don't want to burden the system.

"It got shit done," she said.

Julia can't know for certain what impact posting to X had on Angelina's care. However, she is certain that the posts generated stories in the national media and have been viewed more than one million times. Julia has since heard stories from countless other patients who have suffered because of long ER waits.

"They didn't know how to advocate in the system, and you shouldn't need to," she told me, her frustration still raw. "That's why we have a healthcare system—so the people whose bodies are not okay can have a system which knows how to fix that. Patients shouldn't need to be their own advocate."

In the end, it turned out that Angelina's appendix was not ruptured. Her surgery was successful. She went back to school the week following her surgery and was fully recovered six weeks later. She still plans to become a nurse. Julia says that Angelina had "fantastic follow-up care from the hospitals." Angelina has also had the opportunity to speak about her experience with hospital leadership and Sylvia Jones, then the provincial minister of health.

"I think those made her feel a bit vindicated," says Julia. "That's not an opportunity most people get in the system!"

I salute Julia for effective advocacy in not one but two ERs. Still, I wonder if posting on X or TikTok might become essential to getting care for a loved one. I worry that people who aren't as savvy as Julia will fall even further behind in the queue.

9:55 p.m.

Linus and I hunch over a wide counter in the ambulatory zone to get a closer look at the computer monitor.

"Is that it?" Linus points to a tiny bit of grey haziness on the X-ray of Anabel's foot.

"Yes, that's it." Renata, the medical radiation technologist, or MRT for short, has overheard Linus and stops to admire the X-ray she's taken. She's been taking X-rays about as long as I've worked in the ER.

I zoom in until my nose is six inches from the monitor. "Let's pull up the AP view," I ask.

Renata gently pats Linus's hand away from the keyboard and opens every view of the foot she has carefully taken. She says to him, "You haven't identified the precise location of a glass fragment until you see it in two views."

I smile at Renata. "It helps when a smart MRT superimposes a flat piece of metal in the shape of an arrow that just happens to point to the location of that shard of glass."

"I knew you'd notice." She returns the smile as she walks away.

Linus says, "It looks like the shard is about a centimetre underneath and slightly lateral to the break in Anabel's skin."

"It's definitely reachable with a curved hemostat," I tell him. A curved hemostat looks like a pair of curved scissors, but instead of sharp blades, the curved pieces are interlocking forceps. The handles lock together with a ratchet mechanism. It's an instrument that has other uses besides clamping blood vessels.

Linus grabs a surgical tray that contains instruments and sterile drapes, a vial of local anesthetic, needles, a syringe and two pairs of sterile surgical gloves.

"Sorry it's taken so long," I tell Anabel as she hops up onto a stretcher. "We found the glass. If you agree, I'll disinfect the skin over the top of your foot where the glass is embedded. Next, I'll inject some local to anesthetize the skin. Then I'll use a surgical instrument to hopefully retrieve the glass fragment."

"Go for it," says Anabel, still maintaining her positive attitude after spending more than half a day in the ER.

I don sterile gloves and paint the skin around the cut with a chlorhexidine lollipop to disinfect it.

"Here comes the local," I tell her as I inject it very slowly. "You may feel a bit of burning."

"I hardly felt a thing," she tells me. "That's better than the dentist."

I marvel at Anabel's demeanour. "For someone who has waited as long as you have, you are a fountain of kindness and patience."

"Don't forget, I know a fair bit about what it's like to be healthcare providers at a time like this."

"Let me know if you feel that." I gently poke at the anesthetized skin with the curved hemostat.

"I feel slight pressure but no sharp pain," she replies.

All I can think right now is that my mission stands a good chance of failure unless I can actually retrieve the shard. "Let's hope that I find it and it wants to come out," I say.

"You'll get it," Anabel assures me.

For a moment, I close my eyes and try to conjure up the image on the X-rays. Then I insert the tips of the hemostat into the open cut. Slowly, I inch the instrument lateral to the wound, going millimetre by millimetre and using the hemostat to probe for the glass. Suddenly, the instrument comes up against something hard and makes a scratchy sound.

"I think I felt it," I say hopefully. "Let's see if I can pull it out."

To do that, I retract the closed tips of the hemostat a couple of millimetres. Next, I open the hemostat so that the tips are 3 or 4 millimetres apart. Then I insert it a few millimetres deeper, until I think the tips surround the glass shard.

"Here goes nothing," I say as I close the tips of the hemostat. They make a wonderful scrunching sound, and I can feel them tighten around the shard and lock with a distinct click.

Slowly and gently, I pull out the closed hemostat until I can see that the tips have made purchase around a 2 millimetre shard of pointy glass.

"Hard to believe a teensy little piece of glass like that could cause so much discomfort," I tell Anabel.

"I knew you'd get it."

"Believe me, it doesn't always go that way." I feel a great sense of relief.

There were good options had I not retrieved the glass. Foreign bodies made of organic material—for example, fish bones or wood slivers—should be removed as soon as possible because they can fester. Since glass is inorganic, there is no urgent requirement to remove fragments. And I have on numerous occasions failed to remove glass and other foreign bodies and have had to refer the patient to a specialist's outpatient clinic.

But Anabel had waited close to ten hours for a chance at immediate relief. I felt guilty about how long she had waited for a relatively trivial reason. Had she left the department no better off, I would have felt even worse.

"Here's a little souvenir." I hand her a sterile container with the tiny piece of glass inside.

For some patients, a good outcome makes everything worth the wait.

CHAPTER FIVE

THE LONG HALL

10:20 p.m.

"ER physicians, huddle in the triage area." Cynthia's voice on the intercom sounds edgy. I scribble some orders on a patient's chart as I walk to triage from the farthest end of the waiting room. Tawny and Fix have already arrived.

"Good evening, colleagues." Samir, the night shift doctor, hot-foots it from the hallway where the ER holds patients who are still being cared for by paramedics, clutching four charts. He's the newest hire in the ER, and the most eager to please. Like me, he got called in early to deal with the high volume of patients.

"How are you guys making out?" Cynthia asks a question instead of barking an order. There's an unwritten rule in healthcare culture that nurses don't issue orders to doctors. Instead, they hint.

Erin Sullivan is a doctor friend of mine who worked for five years as a registered nurse before going to medical school. She told me that what she refers to as "nurse-speak" is an oblique form of communicating with doctors. "I would say it's using code and indirect language to communicate a point that [the nurses] feel they can't make overtly."

Nurse-speak has to be subtle and non-confrontational, Erin explained. For example, in her nursing days, she might have found herself assisting a resident who was doing a medical procedure in a way she found both incorrect and potentially dangerous. On a medical procedural show like *Grey's Anatomy*, the nurse might exclaim, "Keep doing that and you'll kill the patient!" Erin says the nurse-speak version of that warning is, "I've never seen the procedure done like that before." The hope is that the inexperienced resident will take the hint and either ask the nurse how to do the procedure correctly or find a more experienced resident or attending physician to help.

Cynthia's polite "How are you guys making out?" is nurse-speak for "Pick up the pace!" She is also asking if we need to call in another doctor to help plough through the patient backlog.

As part of the hospital's contractual agreement with the province to provide emergency services twenty-four hours a day, we post a daily on-call schedule. We need to have physicians on call so they can step in for colleagues who are injured or ill and unable to work. (Absences have been much more frequent since the early days of Covid, when hospitals adopted stricter rules forbidding frontline healthcare workers from coming to work when ill.) We also need to be able to summon additional doctors to work when wait times are getting longer and there are more patients than the scheduled staff can handle. But there are no hard-and-fast rules for exactly when that point is reached. Many ER physicians, including me, are reluctant to ask the doctor on call to come to work because they're embarrassed that they can't keep up with the volume of patients. (My anecdotal experience is that female physicians are more likely to summon the on-call physician because they set aside their own misgivings for the good of the ER.)

I tell the others, "I've seen four patients, and I don't feel like I'm making a dent in the number waiting to be seen."

"Me too," says Tawny. "I'm getting bogged down sorting out the patients I picked up before Brian got here."

"I've got the ambulatory zone under control," says Fix. "I can circle back to the waiting room to see if I can sort out some patients and send them on their way."

"You've been here the longest," I remind him. "I appreciate the help, but please feel free to cherry-pick patients you think you can see in the least amount of time. When you've had enough, hand over what you've got so you can get home to your family."

"Samir, you've just arrived," says Cynthia. "What do you think?"

"I've seen four and I'm just getting started," he says with a big grin on his face. I marvel at his energy.

"Let's review in an hour," I tell the others. "Cynthia, is that a plan?"

"Okay for now." She sounds more hopeful than convinced.

10:30 p.m.

Ahu calls me on my cellphone. "I'm not quite sure what's going on but I'm kind of concerned about my patient."

"I'll meet you in RAZ," I reply, referring to the rapid assessment zone. It's a zone inside the ER for patients deemed stable and not suspected of having life-threatening conditions. The big idea behind RAZ is to assess, treat and discharge such patients as quickly as possible. Ahu's expressed concern for Britany, her twenty-four-year-old patient, gets my attention. Like all residents, Ahu lacks experience, but having worked with her on several shifts, I've learned to take her assessments seriously. Mere months from becoming a full-fledged family doctor, she's starting to make sound clinical judgments without my help. We're a team, and Ahu is my eyes and ears.

When I arrive at RAZ, I see Britany sitting on a stretcher in a cubicle and Ahu waiting for me in a hallway nearby.

"Britany has had pain in her mid-epigastrium for the past three days," Ahu tells me, looking at her notes as we confer. "She says the pain radiates straight through to her back. It was intermittent at first but then became more constant. Last night, it woke her up."

"What's your clinical assessment?"

"Could be a peptic ulcer or gallstones," she says. "But the fact the pain radiates to her back makes me think she's got pancreatitis."

To me, that's plausible. The stomach sits on top of the pancreas in the upper part of the abdomen, so in both conditions Ahu is considering, patients feel pain in roughly the same location. Peptic ulcer is the more common diagnosis. Pancreatitis, which means the pancreas is inflamed, causes more severe pain and is more serious.

The pancreas does two main things: It secretes enzymes that help digest food into the small intestine, and it makes the insulin and glucagon that control blood sugar. In its milder form, acute pancreatitis has a mortality rate of less than one per cent. Its more severe form carries a death rate of between 10 and 30 per cent.

"Britany, I've brought the boss to meet you," Ahu tells her patient.

"Hi, Britany, I'm Dr. Goldman." I note that she's lowering her eyebrows and squeezing her eyelids just slightly. These are signs of acute distress. "Do you want something for the pain?"

"I tried Tylenol and it didn't work," she says. "I'd rather not have any strong pain relievers."

"Is that what made you want to come to the ER now?" I ask as I begin pressing on her upper abdomen.

"That really hurts." Britany's big eyes grow wider as her thin upper lip forms a grimace. Both her upper lip and her nose appear abnormally thin. I've noticed it. That's all I can say at this point.

There is something about her physical appearance that may be a clue to a much more serious medical problem.

"Britany has never had gallstones," says Ahu. "She has one or two glasses of wine per week."

"That's good information," I tell Ahu. The two most common causes of acute pancreatitis are gallstones and excess alcohol use. That Britany has neither makes me wonder if we should look for another diagnosis.

I put some conducting goop on my ultrasound probe and connect it to my phone. Then I hold it out to Ahu. "Want to give it a try?"

She takes the probe with a slight smile on her face. "This will feel a bit cold and gooey," she tells Britany. "It might also be a bit uncomfortable."

Ahu presses the probe onto the midline of her patient's belly near the top, angling it until I get a nice view of a perfectly round black circle surrounded by a white border.

"That's the aorta," says Ahu.

Keeping the aorta in the centre of the phone screen, she inches the probe down the middle of Britany's abdomen until she reaches her belly button. There, the aorta splits into right and left iliac arteries that supply blood to the legs.

"What's the diameter of a normal aorta?" I ask Ahu.

"Two centimetres, or two hashmarks on the scale at the side of the screen," she answers. "Her aorta is of normal diameter throughout the abdomen."

"What does that mean?" Britany asks.

"It means you don't have an aneurysm, or a balloon-like bulge, in your aorta," Ahu replies. "The aorta is a big artery that comes off the heart and runs through the middle of your belly."

"Ahu," I interrupt, "do you mind slowly running the probe back up Britany's abdomen? I thought I saw something."

Ahu slides the probe upwards along the middle of the abdomen.

"Stop right there," I say. "Do you mind if I take the probe for a moment?" As I slowly rock the probe up and down in the upper part of Britany's abdomen just below her diaphragm, a white line running across the aorta appears and disappears.

"What's that?" Ahu asks.

"I'm not sure," I tell my resident. "Britany, that white line may be nothing or it may be something important. We need to do a CT scan of your belly and inject some contrast, or dye, to see if there's anything abnormal inside the aorta. At the same time, we can also check to see if your pancreas is inflamed. One way or another, we're going to find the cause of your pain."

I start to walk out of the room, but Ahu doesn't follow.

"There's something I forgot to ask you," she says to her patient. "Are you double-jointed?"

"You mean like this?" Britany uses her right thumb and forefinger to extend her left thumb until the nail is touching her forearm.

"I'd say you are!" I tell Britany.

As Ahu and I walk to the nearby nursing station to order the scan at a computer terminal, I tell her I'm impressed with her clinical acumen. "Not every resident is as dialed in as you are at this point in your training." Scan ordered, Ahu and I head back to the triage area in search of Cynthia.

"We're concerned about Britany in RAZ," I tell the team leader once we find her. "We think she might be unstable. Is there any chance we can get her in a room?"

RAZ is a high-turnover area of the ER, and patients are whisked into cubicles just long enough to be assessed. Britany, however, is potentially sick enough that she needs to be in a room where she can stay.

"We've got one available stretcher in resus," Cynthia says. "I'd like to keep that open in case the paramedics bring us someone who needs it more urgently. But I might have a stretcher in the hallway," she adds. "Best I can do."

"I appreciate it."

"Shouldn't Britany be in the resuscitation room?" Ahu asks me as we walk away.

"In theory, yes," I reply. "But there are virtually no empty beds and we can't stop the flow of new patients. The nurses are wise to want to keep one stretcher available in case the paramedics bring in a code blue or an unstable patient."

"The next unstable patient could be Britany," says Ahu. "I hope that white line on the ultrasound is nothing."

"Me too."

That the least bad option is a stretcher in a hallway shows just how stressed things have become in ERs across Canada. Most of my career, I've been fortunate to work in ERs that keep hallway patients to a minimum and hold them there for the smallest possible number of hours. But at one ER in Prince Edward Island, hallway patients are depressingly routine.

Dr. Trevor Jain is an accomplished ER physician who is also an expert in disaster medicine and the director of the paramedicine program at the University of Prince Edward Island in Charlottetown. When I asked him how he felt his island ER was functioning, he told me, "A senior nursing leader told me that this year the emergency department is the largest inpatient unit in our hospital." He added that the hospital where he works typically has about thirty patients who have been admitted but are kept in the ER because there are no beds available on the wards.

The time some patients stay in Jain's ER is mind-boggling. "It wouldn't be unusual for me to go in and see three or four patients who have been on stretchers for a week," he said. "I've seen patients stay twelve or fourteen days. There's one patient that was in there for three weeks. Some of those patients can have their entire hospital stay in the emergency department and literally be discharged as an inpatient from the emergency department." He's convinced that PEI has it worse than other provinces. "When we see in other provinces that patients stay in the ER for three days," he said, "we kind of roll our eyes."

Certain kinds of patients are more likely than others to remain in an ER hallway without getting a bed upstairs. In many hospitals, for example, a lack of psychiatric beds means patients with mental health crises are more likely to get stuck in the ER. Jain said that in his hospital, older patients with dementia sometimes remain in the ER for days, in part because of a lack of frontline nurses and other factors unique to the hospital where he works. "In order for us to get our patients to the floors, they have to meet certain criteria," he explained. "If the patient has dementia and wanders or is at risk for falling, these are barriers to getting that patient admitted to the floor."

Like other hospitals across Canada, the one where Jain works is also grappling with a severe lack of long-term care beds in the province. Of 229 acute care hospital beds, at any one time as many as 50 are occupied by patients waiting for nursing homes and who are not ill enough to need a hospital to look after them. And PEI has an additional factor that makes ERs there more prone to hallway medicine. "I think it's different because we're so small," he told me. He noted that compared with other provinces, PEI has more administrative personnel who decide policies, including how hospital and long-term care beds are used. "We have a lot of frustration on the front line because we don't understand why we can't pivot and improve the system just one or two per cent."

Talking about bureaucracy makes it seem as if having patients in the hallway for days and even weeks at a time is just an inconvenience. Jain stressed that's not the case. "Every day, we're dangerously overcrowded because we have patients that are waiting to go to stretchers in the hospital . . . and the nursing ratios are horrific," he explained. "Patients are not getting the care they need."

Here's how the Canadian Association of Emergency Physicians described the ramifications of hallway medicine in its 2024 publication *EM:POWER: The Future of Emergency Care*: "Hospital inpatients deteriorate if held for hours or days on hard narrow ED [emergency department] stretchers in crowded noisy rooms without privacy, bathroom access, or sleep, and where the lights never go out. Acutely ill arrivals with strokes and miscarriages languish or deteriorate in ED waiting rooms when stretchers are blocked by inpatients."

In 2024, NHS England, which oversees the National Health Service in that country, produced guidance on "providing safe and good quality care in temporary escalation spaces." Emergency doctors took NHS England to task for apparently suggesting that hallway medicine can be delivered safely. The guidance was roundly condemned by the Royal College of Emergency Medicine. RCEM president Dr. Adrian Boyle told *The Independent*, "While we understand why this guidance has been issued, as a College we are concerned that it represents a normalisation of what is an unacceptable and dangerous situation."

"We do know that mortality or morbidity skyrockets," said Jain. "Any emergency physician should not be scared to say that, because that's the truth in every overcrowded emergency department in Canada. We're seeing adverse outcomes."

On top of everything else, hallway patients aren't receiving the supports that patients receive when they're on an actual admission ward. Admission wards are better than ERs at taking care of admitted patients, Jain said, because they have the resources to look after patients holistically. "We don't have the equipment and staff," he told me. "We don't have occupational and physiotherapy. We have some social work but not full outpatient social work. We don't have pharmacy medication checks."

And this is all happening on a huge and ever-increasing scale. As CAEP succinctly put it, "The wrong patient in the wrong place on a large scale generates inefficiency, system cost, and adverse patient outcomes."

Admitted patients in the ER are the wrong patients in the wrong place. But in an ER not far from PEI, they have plenty of the right patients in the wrong place too.

Picture a long, skinny department broken down into five nursing pods, each with a nursing station and some rooms around it. A hallway encircles the whole department like a great big racetrack. In that hallway are six stretchers filled with patients who are cared for by a nurse and a paramedic who works for the hospital. Around the corner from those six stretchers is another hallway that can hold as many as twenty stretchers filled with patients at any given time.

That's how Halifax doctor Lorri Beatty describes the hallway where she sees the majority of her ER patients on a typical night shift. This is ER hallway medicine on steroids.

Beatty, a twelve-year veteran of the ER, said she and her colleagues now face the near-nightly grind of trying to find a private place to assess patients fully. "One night," she told me, "we had a patient with really bad psychosis who was very agitated and at risk to themselves and others, and who needed medical sedation like an injection to help them calm down." She remembered that there was a little room not far from the hallway area that had a photocopier, some nursing desks and other things. It was the only private place left in the ER, and that's where the patient was taken.

"Into this room with a photocopier and desks and chairs, to be restrained on a stretcher and given medication to calm down because there was no other place," she recalled. "I don't think I'm exaggerating, but the next day all the desks and the photocopier were gone from that room. The door was taken off and a curtain was hung up and suddenly, it's a patient care space." To this day, this little space is where hallway patients are taken should privacy be needed. It's not ideal, but at least it can be closed off a bit "so you can talk to them and do a physical exam while preserving some degree of their privacy."

The thing is, once that bonus space is filled up, it's back to the hallway. "It was recognized probably a year and a half ago that this is not going away," Beatty noted with some frustration. "We are now going to be giving people the entirety of their ED stay in the hallway."

For patients arriving by ambulance, that stay in the hallway does not begin officially until paramedics have offloaded them to an ER stretcher and handed them over to a nurse. Until then—in Nova Scotia as in other provinces—paramedics must continue caring for the patients they bring in.

Offload delay is not a new problem in Nova Scotia. It has been talked about in that province for years. These days, however, a nursing shortage in ERs has exacerbated the issue, meaning paramedics must wait even longer to offload their patients. ER closures across Nova Scotia, as in other provinces, mean more crowded regional emergency departments and more delays. There's also attrition in the ranks of paramedics brought on by retirements, stress leave and the lure of more pay and better working conditions in other provinces. These factors create frustration for the people who work in Nova Scotia ERs and their patients. They also reduce the number of paramedics available to respond to emergencies.

To get ambulance crews back on the road, paramedics in offload delay may be asked to keep watch over two patients at a time.

In the ER where Dr. Lorri Beatty works, that means there may be as many as ten pairs of paramedics looking after twenty patients in the hallway. These patients may be in offload delay, but they're not out of sight and out of mind. Beatty and her colleagues are responsible for their welfare as well as that of the thirty or so ER patients who have been offloaded.

"You come in at 10 p.m. and end up having to take handover"—the transfer of patients from one physician to another—"on almost the entire department, which now includes those same thirty beds, plus six in the offload zone plus up to twenty patients in the ambulance hallway," she said. "So you're taking handover on this enormous volume of patients and you're expected to kind of continue caring for all of them through the shift and collect handover from the three different docs who are going home at midnight, and still see all the new patients who are coming in, and manage a medical student or resident if you have a learner. It's such an enormous burden right now that the fun of the medicine . . . is sort of counterbalanced by the burden."

As for the patients whose stretchers drape the hallways, Beatty says she has to make a snap decision whether to take a history and forgo a physical or ferry them to and from the patient room that used to house the photocopy machine to do a more complete physical examination.

"Not that long ago this woman came in who was pretty sick and it wasn't really clear why," she recalled. "She made some passing comments about hemorrhoids. I couldn't figure out why this lady was so sick and getting sicker." Beatty decided to move her down to the photocopy room for a physical that included a rectal examination. "I found that she had this big, terrible infection on her backside which I totally could have missed and not ever diagnosed." Beatty's instincts possibly saved the patient, who ended up in the operating room for surgical drainage of an abscess.

Beatty's instincts have been honed over her dozen years working in the ER. But she can't be everywhere all the time in the busy emergency department where she plies her trade.

She told me the story of a young adult who had come to the ER with intestinal bleeding. The cause of the bleeding was an arteriovenous malformation, or AVM, of the small intestine, which is an abnormality on the inner lining of the bowel wall. Roughly 5 per cent of all gastrointestinal bleeding comes from the small bowel, and AVMs cause 30 to 40 per cent of bleeds. AVMs are a common cause of bleeding in patients over the age of fifty, though cancers, polyps, Crohn's disease and ulcers are also common causes. When bleeding from the small bowel is a tiny trickle, it causes anemia, which leads to fatigue and shortness of breath. When the bleeding is brisk, it causes a hemorrhage. Blood from the small intestine is usually dark red or a shade of maroon that looks like port wine. Beatty said the patient had arrived at the ER earlier in the day and was sent home after being observed for several hours. At home, the bleeding started up again, and paramedics brought the patient back to the hospital.

In Nova Scotia, the emergency response for the entire province is run by Emergency Health Services, or EHS. Paramedic crews are dispatched through a central communications centre in Dartmouth. When large numbers of Halifax-based paramedics are taking care of patients in offload delay in local ERs, EHS makes up for the shortfall by dispatching crews from outside of Halifax. "It was a night where there were no beds in the department to offload EHS patients, and the patient was picked up by an out-of-town crew that wasn't used to hallway medicine," Beatty remembered. "Most of the paramedics that work in Halifax are used to spending a good chunk of their shift sitting with patients in hallways. They've learned over time how to assess and reassess and monitor patients and take care of them because they've been forced to do it."

Beatty said that when local paramedics are worried about a patient, they watch them more vigilantly. They keep them on a heart monitor, check the blood pressure regularly and monitor the patient's oxygen saturation. But the paramedics taking care of the young woman that night weren't used to closely monitoring patients in the hallway.

"By the time I got to see this person in the hallway, the paramedic gave a report about what happened and said, 'The patient has been sleeping ever since arriving.'" Beatty said the paramedic's description didn't track with what she could see plainly. "The patient was very pale and kind of sweaty," Beatty explained. She quickly realized that the woman was not stable and sleeping but was in severe shock from acute blood loss. "The [systolic] blood pressure was 60 [millimetres mercury], which is not in keeping with life. And then we had a quick peek under the sheet: The whole stretcher underneath was pooled with blood."

Faced with a life-threatening crisis in a patient far too young to be bleeding to death right under their noses, Beatty and the nurses sprang into action. "We got that patient into a room pretty quick," she said. "I didn't care if there was a room. We just turfed the least sick person into the hallway." From that point, the resuscitation went smoothly. "When you have a proper space to care for someone, the ER team works really well. The nurses got good IV access, and we were able to start massive transfusions."

Beatty summoned the senior resident on call for general surgery stat. That the resident came quickly was instrumental in helping save the patient's life. "We were able to resuscitate this person back to consciousness and stabilize her well enough that we were able to get her to the operating room." In the OR, surgeons were able to find the AVM and remove the bleeding section of intestine. What they didn't know until they saw for themselves was whether the bowels on either side of the removed section were healthy enough to be attached to one another. If not, the patient would need an ostomy bag to collect bowel movements quite possibly for the rest of her life. Fortunately, despite everything the patient had endured, the surrounding intestines looked pink and healthy. Surgeons were able to stitch them together so that an ostomy was not needed.

"That felt like a win," said Beatty. "We actually did something good for a patient that night."

Beatty's patient reminds me of Molly, the woman with the ruptured ectopic pregnancy who we brought in from the waiting room in the nick of time. We relish talking about near misses when we manage to save them.

But Dr. Trevor Jain, the ER physician in PEI, says it's important to remember that not every patient who languishes for hours or days in a hallway has a good outcome. "I am tired of folks saying, 'Well, nobody died,'" Jain complained. "That's not good enough. That should not be the benchmark for the care that Canadians get in the emergency department."

Unfortunately, hallway patients and hallway deaths go hand in hand. And not just in Atlantic Canada.

Dr. Kashif Pirzada is an emergency doctor who works at some of Toronto's busiest ERs. One of them sees three hundred to four hundred patients a day. "I think there's a breaking point," Pirzada told me. "I had a case I talked about on a TV interview where someone was waiting seven hours on an EMS stretcher. They were diagnosed with pneumonia and not doing well." Pirzada said the person did eventually get offloaded onto one of the stretchers in the ER, but an hour later, the patient went into cardiac arrest and died.

"Could we have done something in those seven hours to reverse that?" asked Pirzada. "Could we have given fluids, and antibiotics? Maybe not, but that person deserved that chance, right?"

According to figures obtained by the Nova Scotia NDP caucus through a freedom of information request and shared with CBC News, 180 patients died in ERs across the province in the fourth quarter of 2022. Thirty-two of those deaths occurred in the last two weeks of 2022 alone. Two in particular prompted the province to announce a plan to provide faster care for urgent patients. On December 31, 2022, thirty-seven-year-old Allison Holthoff of Tidnish died of cardiac arrest in the ER at Cumberland Regional Health Care Centre in Amherst after waiting more than six hours to be seen by a physician. A day earlier, sixty-seven-year-old Charlene Snow, who had left the ER of a hospital in Cape Breton after waiting roughly seven hours, died at home of fluid build-up in her heart.

Holthoff's death triggered a review—required by the province's Quality-improvement Information Protection Act—of the circumstances surrounding her care in hospital. The Nova Scotia Health Authority, which operates the province's hospitals and which completed the review, told the *Halifax Examiner* in April 2023 that it was unwilling to share the recommendations with anyone other than Allison's husband, Günter Holthoff. A statement of claim has been filed on behalf of Holthoff's husband and her three children.

Dr. Lorri Beatty was one of the key signatories to a letter sent to Nova Scotia Premier Tim Houston in January 2023. In it, dozens of physicians expressed concerns that changes announced by the province to ease the load on ERs—among them, creating doctor-led triage teams to focus on admitting patients more quickly and assigning more physician assistants and nurse practitioners—would not address the underlying problems. Beatty and the other doctors who signed the letter suggested that the focus should be on moving admitted patients stuck in the ER to the wards faster.

"Admitted patients are filling the beds that are needed for paramedics to offload new patients, creating delays in ambulance offload," read the letter. "These beds filled with admitted patients result in overflowing waiting rooms, long waits, fewer ambulances in communities, and ultimately tragic outcomes. Indeed, patients waiting six to eight hours before being admitted to hospital suffer a death rate 8% higher than those who don't wait. In other words, one extra patient death occurs for every three to four days of a blocked ED."

The province subsequently tried to address the issues raised in the letter by hiring non-medical personnel, called patient advocates, to provide people waiting to be seen with comfort measures such as warm blankets and beverages. As well, in an effort to get paramedic crews back on the road faster, the province took a page from Alberta and created "offload zones" where nurses are assigned to care for groups of patients brought to the ER by ambulance.

But Beatty says the patient advocates have not helped the situation and at times have distracted triage nurses by advocating excessively for the patients they see. And as happened in Alberta, ER nurses assigned to offload zones are not new hires; they are taken from the ranks of nurses inside the ER. As a result, beds have to be closed for lack of nurses, thus exacerbating the problem this approach is designed to fix.

Meanwhile, Beatty says the situation at Nova Scotia ERs has actually become worse. "The place has deteriorated so much in the past year," she told me. "Those were the good old days, and I miss when we only had that degree of dysfunction."

11:05 p.m.

Britany is on a stretcher in the hallway. A dose of hydromorphone has improved her physical discomfort, but she has an apprehensive look on her face as a service attendant releases the brake on her stretcher and wheels her to the CT room for her scans.

I'm starting to get into a bit of a rhythm. Samir's early arrival for the night shift means he's now on tap to take on every acutely ill patient inside the ER or in the waiting room. Under normal circumstances, I'd move over to the RAZ to see patients who have been deemed less acutely ill. But according to the plan formulated during our huddle, Tawny has agreed to keep seeing patients in RAZ for a while longer while I pick up a few more of those with major illnesses. For a moment, though, I can relax long enough to do some follow-up. I open the radiology viewing software, key in my password and begin scrolling through a list of patients to see if the radiologists have reported on any of the scans I've ordered.

Soming, the resident in obstetrics and gynecology, catches my eye and walks briskly towards me.

"Molly's heading for the ICU," she tells me, plopping on the countertop beside me with a thud and a sigh. "We gave her eight units of packed red blood cells during surgery. There were more than two litres of blood in her belly."

"I don't know how she survived."

"Her will to live is stronger than her hemoglobin," she says.

"Has any family surfaced?" I ask.

"I've had zero time to look," Soming says. "Tonight, it's the ICU. Assuming she's stable, I think she'll be transferred to the ward in a day or maybe two."

"Any idea how many weeks she was pregnant?"

"The pregnancy that caused all that bleeding was not that large, just eight centimetres long and four centimetres in diameter," she says, holding out her thumb and index finger for dramatic effect. "Just amazing."

"I don't suppose you know much yet about the circumstances of Molly's pregnancy?" I ask.

"Once she's on the ward, we'll get the social worker to ask her about sex partners. We're testing her for HIV and other sexually transmitted infections. We'll see if there's any next of kin."

"Thanks for the update," I tell Soming, "and the save."

"Thank *you* for acting so quickly," she says, then she turns and walks away.

My eyes return to the list of completed X-rays on the computer screen. I find Larry's name and click to read the radiologist's final report. Ahu joins me at the computer.

I read aloud. "'On this contrast-enhanced CT scan, axial views demonstrate multiple nodules localized to the mesogastric and hypogastric areas on the anterior abdominal wall as well as between loops of bowel and throughout the pelvis.'"

"That's not good," says Ahu.

"No," I agree, "it isn't."

All that terse technical jargon comes to a cruel point: Larry has some sort of cancer with extensive metastases inside his belly.

"I have to tell Larry and his wife," I say, pushing back from the terminal.

"Mind if I join you?" Ahu asks. "I haven't handled that many of these conversations. I'd like to see how an experienced physician does it."

"I'd appreciate that," I tell her as we head back to the waiting room.

We find Larry and Helen on the same chairs they were in when we first met.

"Larry, I'm really sorry you and Helen have had to spend hours and hours in the waiting room," I tell them. "I need to bring you back in so I can give you the results of your CT scan."

Larry holds Helen's hand as she slowly and tenderly guides him to the side room and helps him onto the stretcher. My type A personality often leaves me shuddering when patients require extra time to get in and out of rooms and on and off stretchers. But in this moment, I can see the love between them and I know just how important it will be to help them get through the difficult days that lie ahead.

CHAPTER SIX

THE ER IS CLOSED

12:05 a.m.

Brian, can I hand over a patient to you?" asks Fix. "Everybody on my list has either been discharged or referred to a specialist for probable admission."

He has stayed two hours beyond his scheduled departure time. He looks tired, and he's one of the most energetic colleagues I've ever worked with.

When it comes to emergency medicine, patient handovers are a double-edged sword. On one hand, they are fraught with risk—an important detail about the patient's history is missed; some part of the plan to diagnose and treat the problem falls through the cracks. These aren't idle concerns. Handovers can sometimes result in delays in diagnosis and treatment, confusion regarding proper care and increased lengths of stay.

On the other hand, handovers are inevitable given the exigencies and inefficiencies of emergency and hospital medicine. In the final scheduled hour of your shift, you pick up a surprisingly complex patient who requires an extensive and time-consuming workup. Or you see a patient whose back pain or nausea stubbornly refuses to go away so that you can issue a discharge.

"Phil, you need to go home and get some rest," I tell him as he leads me down the hall to a cubicle, where I find a young man lying on a stretcher. Beside him is a young woman who looks concerned.

"Rodrigo, Christine, I'd like you to meet Dr. Goldman," says Phil. "He's taking over for me."

"Glad to know you." I nod to the twosome.

Phil relates his patient's history. "Rodrigo is a thirty-four-year-old male who has gnawing abdominal pain, a change in bowel habits and decreased appetite for the past three weeks. The past two days, he's been nauseated but hasn't vomited. He has no fever."

"He's also been losing weight," Christine chimes in.

"How much?" I ask her.

"Maybe ten kilos."

"How do you know?" Rodrigo asks. "I haven't weighed myself."

"I can tell," she replies, looking straight at me and Phil.

"What's the change in bowel habits?" I ask.

"I'm constipated," says Rodrigo. "My bowel movements look like broken pieces."

"He's been talking like that for two years," Christine interjects. "He also had bleeding."

"My doctor said it's due to hemorrhoids."

"On the physical examination," continues Phil, "his heart rate and blood pressure are normal. His temperature is normal. Head and neck, chest and cardiac exams are normal. His abdomen is soft but he's tender on the left-hand side. No signs of peritonitis. His blood tests are normal."

"What's the plan?" I ask him.

"I've given him injections for pain and for nausea," says Phil. "I ordered a CT scan of his abdomen and pelvis. Radiology has been slow. I ordered the CT four hours ago. It's only being done right now. Sorry it's taken so long, folks."

"Once the CT is done, I'll let you know what the radiologist says," I tell the couple. "Rodrigo, if you have any more pain or nausea, let the nurse know."

"Thanks, Doctor," says Rodrigo.

Phil and I leave the cubicle.

"Can you let me know what the scan shows?" says Phil. "I'm kind of worried about him."

"So am I."

1:00 a.m.

Phil is heading for the exit as Cynthia summons the rest of the emergency physicians back to the triage area for another huddle. Samir is seeing a patient at the near end of the long hall where we stack stretchers brought in by paramedics. They have a look of resignation as they wait to offload their patients to ER nurses. The waiting room is even busier than when I first arrived. There is now a lineup of patients and paramedics waiting to speak to the triage nurses.

Suddenly, the red phone in the triage area rings loudly. The red phone is a hotline that connects the ER to Toronto Paramedic Services (TPS). Nurses, doctors, the extern who takes blood and does ECGs on patients in the waiting room all snap to attention. Even the security guards stop what they're doing.

One ring followed by silence is a false alarm. Two rings means the desk supervisor at TPS wants to speak to the nurse in charge.

A pregnant pause brings a second ring.

Broadly speaking, there are two possible reasons for the call. One is to alert the ER that paramedics are bringing in a patient in extreme distress, often in cardiac arrest. This is why most of us stop what we're doing whenever we hear the red phone. The more common reason is that the desk supervisor wants to complain to the team leader about how long it's taking to offload patients the paramedics have brought in.

Cynthia picks up the phone. "Team leader here," she says.

I never know precisely what Cynthia is thinking. What I do know is that she keeps it all behind a poker face born of years of experience.

"Uh-huh," she tells the desk supervisor in a matter-of-fact tone that makes me grin. She catches the look on my face and puts an index finger to her pursed lips. She's telling me not to do or say anything that might make her chuckle. Her practised technique is to listen first to the supervisor, then give him or her an earful.

"I appreciate your concern," she says finally after two long minutes of respectful silence. "You remember that young woman with agitation you sent us? She's in the recovery room after getting a ruptured ectopic fixed." Now Cynthia smiles at me. "That plus two critically ill patients in heart failure who arrived at nearly the same time, both of whom needed intubation. Plus another patient with an acute stroke who arrived shortly after that. Plus the other fourteen patients you've brought us in the last four hours. You'd *think* we're the only ER that's open."

From the look on Cynthia's face, I'm guessing that the desk supervisor is imploring her (and us) to offload patients more quickly so the paramedic crews can get back on the road.

"We'll do our best," she says before hanging up.

"Nicely done," I tell her. She could have snapped at the supervisor but kept her cool instead. It's an underappreciated skill that the greatest emergency nurses possess.

Samir and Tawny arrive at the triage area.

"Should we call the backup physician?" Cynthia asks.

Samir shakes his head. "I think it's cruel to wake the backup after they've gone to sleep," he says.

"The onslaught has to stop sometime, doesn't it?" I reply.

"Hey, Samir," says Tawny, "I've got a fractured ankle I need to fix. Can you sedate the patient?"

"Sure. Call me when you're ready to go."

As we're about to disperse, Cynthia gives us some bad news:

Stefan, the nurse who has been working in the ambulatory zone, is going home.

"He's back today at 7:30 a.m.," she explains. "He worked sixteen hours straight and needs to get some sleep. It means AZ won't have a nurse until the morning. I'll cover the best I can, but with the way things are out here, I don't think I'll be much help. Think you guys can manage?"

"We have no choice," says Samir.

Stefan and most of the other nurses who work here are pulling lots of overtime these days because Canada is in the grip of a critical nursing shortage decades in the making. A 2012 simulation model by Gail Tomblin Murphy, a registered nurse and chief nurse executive at Nova Scotia Health, concluded that Canada would be short more than 60,000 RNs in 2022 and more than 117,000 by 2030.

A 2024 survey published on the Statista website found that roughly one in four nurses in Canada were considering leaving their current job, with one in ten wanting to leave the profession as a whole. Baby boomer nurses are retiring, and younger nurses are far from satisfied with their work.

Chronic understaffing sets up a vicious cycle. It means that on the wards, in the ICU and in the ER, fewer nurses look after more patients. "Insufficient staffing increases nurse workload to above normal demands and can threaten patient safety," wrote Lisa McKendrick Calder, Leanne Topola and Tanya Heuver from Edmonton's MacEwan University, in a 2024 article in *The Conversation*. It also means that nurses like Stefan are pressed to work more hours per week in overtime and extra shifts. Both of these issues magnify dissatisfaction and set the stage for an even bigger shortfall.

A 2022 report by the Canadian Federation of Nurses Unions says the exodus was well established prior to Covid, though the pandemic made it more acute. "The additional pressures, workload and stress stemming from the pandemic have exacerbated the situation," the report states. "Many nurses are leaving the profession, spurred by worsening working conditions and an increased psychological burden."

In urban ERs across Canada, the nursing shortage often means closing a zone, as Cynthia is forced to do on this night. But in rural and remote parts of the country, the shortfall means shutting down entire ERs and putting communities at risk. That's what happened when the ER at the hospital in Perth, Ontario, shut its doors for nearly four weeks in July 2022. But before we can get to the story of this closure, it's important to explain just how good this ER is.

The formal name is the Perth and Smiths Falls District Hospital, GWM Site. Locals still call it the Great War Memorial Hospital of Perth District. In 1995, the Perth hospital merged with the hospital in Smiths Falls, about a twenty kilometre drive away.

The merger made for a bit of grumbling among physicians in Perth. "When the district needed a CT scanner, it went to Smiths Falls," said one ER doctor. "When it needed an MRI, it went to Smiths Falls." Still, Perth's ER is a gem of a place inside a hospital that punches way above its weight. In 2021, Perth became the first hospital in eastern Ontario, the first community hospital in Canada and just the fifth hospital in Canada to do knee replacements with a system called ROSA, which stands for robotic surgical assistant. ROSA is helping orthopedic surgeons in Perth perform a high volume of joint replacement surgeries with great outcomes. "People are surprised at how many knee replacements we do at our little hospital," one anesthesiologist told me with obvious pride.

On a rainy day in July 2024, Dr. Al Drummond showed me around the emergency department. At seventy, Drummond has a craggy face and a crusty demeanour, but he still exudes a passion for emergency medicine after forty-two years and counting. He calls his ER "small but mighty." It's a modest-looking compact rectangular space with ten stretchers that surround a central nursing station and hub for physicians, but it manages to see 25,000 patients a year.

Emergency medicine was in its infancy when Drummond arrived in Perth in the early 1980s. It was a time when GPs saw patients in their clinics. If people needed emergency care, their doctors met them in the ER to provide it. This wasn't always the best or safest approach, Drummond explained, because it sometimes resulted in substandard care from doctors who hadn't kept up with advances in emergency medicine. "It wasn't fair to either the physician or the patient," he told me.

As medical director, Drummond made "the personal commitment" to recruit and train doctors to practise emergency medicine as a specialty. "If you were going to work in the emergency department, then you were going to fully commit to maintaining skills." He brought in standardized training programs like Advanced Cardiovascular Life Support and Advanced Trauma Life Support, as well as courses in airway management. He made sure to include emergency nurses in the courses he arranged. He also sought feedback on the care his team was providing from larger hospitals in Ottawa and Kingston, where his small ER frequently transferred patients.

"And lucky for me, I guess everybody kind of bought into the program," Drummond said. "It could have backfired. It could have blown up in my face. You know, five of the eight doctors could have said, 'Fuck you, we're not doing this.' I would have been up the creek. But they didn't. They all bought in and did their very best." Drummond lifted the ER by its bootstraps until its outcomes were as good as those of the best teaching hospitals in Canada. Along the way, he helped bring together a core group of physicians who practise emergency medicine at a high level and have family practices in the community.

One of those is Dr. Anil Kuchinad. Originally from London, Ontario, Kuchinad completed a master's in neuroscience in the field of chronic pain and interned in South Africa for the Canadian International Development Agency before returning to Canada for medical school at the University of Toronto. He did a residency in family medicine at McGill University before settling down with his wife, Kathryn, in Perth.

That was ten years ago. He says he's glad he and his wife decided to stay.

"I think it's an excellent collaborative group of people," he told me, noting that the ER physicians teach residents and medical students. When I visited, the ER was hosting first-year medical students from the University of Ottawa. They don't see patients but shadow the physicians so they can get a sense of what it's like to practise ER medicine in a smaller hospital.

"We have a well-run emergency department with a critical mass of physicians," Kuchinad told me, explaining that colleagues are willing to come in on a moment's notice to help cope with high volumes of patients or major incidents like serious car accidents with multiple casualties. He also said that the doctors support each other to a degree that isn't always possible at ERs in smaller communities. On the day I was there, one of the doctors had dislocated her thumb in a pickup hockey game. "She needs four ER shifts covered urgently," Kuchinad said. "I'm filling in for her on a last-minute basis. Another doctor coming in today is a physician who doesn't work a lot of emergency room medicine but is willing to help because this is an SOS call." They go the extra mile because they respect each other. "We're good local friends and not just colleagues. I feel well supported here in terms of my group."

After showing me around the ER, Drummond took me on a tour of the rest of the hospital. Like the ER, it's compact—just four floors. Although Drummond is often direct, it was clear to me that he had an easy rapport with everyone he worked with.

Upstairs, he introduced me to Tiggy, a nurse who had been in the ER for nearly fourteen years but recently left to work on the rehabilitation ward. "Tiggy is one of our most senior, experienced and dedicated emergency nurses," Drummond said, before adding with a grin, "who I'm sad to say is now rotting away up here."

The respect and affection between Drummond and Tiggy, whose full name is Tegan Baker, was obvious. "Al is lovely," she said. "He and I are like soul people. We say how it is. We're honest. You may not like it, but that's what it is. He has a good heart and he loves to help."

Tiggy said that she fell in love with the ER the moment she arrived and is proud of the patients she helped save. She told me about one time early in her ER career when she and her doctor colleagues worked on a pregnant woman who was on her way to the hospital to give birth when the car her husband was driving was struck head-on by an intoxicated driver. The woman was thrown through the windshield.

"She was covered in glass," Tiggy recalled. "Her entire face had been degloved." This is the term doctors use for an injury in which the skin is peeled away from its underlying bones, muscles and nerves. "All you could see was her skeleton." Incredibly, despite her youth and inexperience, Tiggy was able to keep her composure and be there for the woman. "We cleaned her face off and timed her contractions," she told me. "I just remember telling her not to open her eyes," to spare the woman the shock of seeing her own face. Eventually, they transferred her to the Ottawa Hospital, where she gave birth. She also required extensive facial plastic surgery.

Fast-forward seven years, and a woman appeared at the nurses' station in the ER and asked if her name was Tiggy.

"I saw this faint scar on the woman's face and instantly recognized her as the woman who had that dreadful injury . . . She said she'd been looking for me. She recognized my voice from across the room. She said I'd kept her calm during such a tragic event. And the son she gave birth to in the wake of the accident is seven years old."

What made that rescue so special to Tiggy was not the medicine but the human connection. "I've delivered babies in the back of an ambulance, and that's exciting," she told me. "But to have somebody who could never remember your face and had no idea what you looked like come and thank you for helping her feel calm in such a stressful experience is really nice."

With such deep and meaningful memories of her time in the emergency department, I had to wonder why Tiggy left. We'll get to that part of the story in a bit because it's critical for understanding why this scrappy little ER was forced to close its doors for nearly a month.

As Drummond and I left Tiggy to her patients in the rehabilitation ward, I remarked that there seemed to be something uniquely special about the culture of the ER in Perth and the spirit of the people who work there.

"This *is* a unique place," agreed Drummond, who told me he'd worked in nearby communities like Pembroke, Hawkesbury and Carleton Place before coming to Perth. "The hospital is an integral part of healthcare provision in the community," he said, noting that the town has become a destination for retired people, and those people often have complicated medical conditions to manage, such as diabetes, obesity, chronic obstructive pulmonary disease and heart disease. "It's extremely well regarded by the people who live here. They depend on us."

James Keelaghan certainly does. The sixty-four-year-old singer-songwriter is one of Canada's most successful and prolific musicians. He won his first Juno Award in 1994 and was nominated for the Traditional Roots Album of the Year for his latest album, *Second Hand*, in 2024. Keelaghan has a knack for writing songs about historical events that still resonate today, like the internment of

Japanese Canadians during the Second World War, or the FLQ crisis. Since 2018, he has been the artistic director of the Stewart Park Festival in Perth, and he's also served as the artistic director of the Summerfolk Music and Crafts Festival in Owen Sound, Ontario. In 2023, he spent three hundred days on the road performing.

In March 2024, at around ten on a Tuesday morning, he was sitting in his modest home in Perth when he experienced the universal emotion of deathly fear from an illness that is all too common. "I started to feel pressure on the left side of my chest," he recalled. "Then I got incredible pain in my jaw. I'm having a heart attack."

This being rural Ontario, Keelaghan wasn't sure that his heart could wait long enough for an ambulance. He put on his coat, grabbed his wallet and headed for his van to drive to the ER, which is four minutes away by car. Once there, he walked up a little hill and told the admitting clerk he was having a heart attack. He was placed on a stretcher, where a nurse took an ECG.

"I remember the nurse turning his head and his mouth opening and then the room just filled up with people," Keelaghan told me. The nurses gave him two baby Aspirins and a dose of Plavix, both blood-thinning medications that reduce the amount of heart damage and the risk of death. He was also given morphine to ease his chest pain.

He asked a nurse what was going on.

"Well, you're in fact having a heart attack," she replied.

"Is it serious?" he asked her. "She looked at me like I was an idiot and just said, 'It's a heart attack.'"

Fortunately for Keelaghan, there was a paramedic crew waiting in the ER's driveway. The doctors and nurses immediately transferred the folksinger onto a stretcher and into the ambulance, and after that, it was lights and sirens all the way to the University of Ottawa Heart Institute. The UOHI is one of Canada's largest cardiac centres. It cares for more than 100,000 patients each year and offers everything from prevention and diagnosis to treatment, rehabilitation, research and education.

Keelaghan told me that as soon as he arrived at UOHI, he was rushed into an angiography suite, where an interventional cardiologist injected contrast dye into his coronary arteries. "Sure enough, doctors found a blockage," he said. "They put in a stent. At 1:00 p.m. I was up in a hospital bed recovering."

The total elapsed time from onset of chest pain to recovery following angioplasty was less than three hours. Keelaghan still can't believe that he was able to get from a country ER to an advanced urban cardiac institute so quickly. As an urban ER physician, I frankly can't believe that the ER in Perth gets results like that.

Keelaghan still needs two more stents, but his health is on the upswing. "I am feeling better than I have in years," he told me. "Way more energy. It's a new lease on life."

For Al Drummond, who until he retired recently was Keelaghan's family doctor, this is how they roll in the Perth ER. "We have gone to great lengths to position ourselves as a reliable partner in a system of care—be it trauma, cardiac or stroke," he explained. "Jim's story suggests that it can work very well."

That's what you get when the ER in Perth is open. Which only makes its prolonged closure all the more disturbing.

On July 1, 2022, the Perth and Smiths Falls District Hospital board announced that the ER in Perth would close the next day, a Saturday, and remain closed until the following Thursday. The shutdown took place during the seventh wave of the Covid pandemic. At the time, the World Health Organization was reporting that 566,631,276 people worldwide had been infected with Covid and

6,390,389 had died of it. Public Health Ontario was reporting close to 1,000 hospitalizations in the province, with 118 patients in intensive care and 48 on ventilators. For frontline healthcare providers, there was no relief from a pandemic that was then in its third year.

Townspeople reacted to the board's announcement with shock. Even people supposedly in the know—like Ed McPherson, a retired paramedic and Perth town councillor—were caught off guard.

"I had no idea," McPherson told me. "I received a phone call from our mayor, who said a private confidential letter had gone out from the [hospital] board to the members of council and to the physicians that the hospital was going to close the emergency room. None of us saw this coming. It was something you didn't anticipate. We never envisioned that the hospital would actually close its emergency room."

Dr. Al Drummond said the original plan was to have the ER close its doors each night at 11:00. The thinking in provincial government circles was that small hospitals like the one in Perth treat a small number of patients whose conditions aren't that complex. The assumption was that it would be relatively safe to close the ER at night. "Across the country, you hear that repeatedly: 'For low volume and low acuity, we can substitute a nurse practitioner or a paramedic.'" That idea was bad enough, Drummond thought, but somehow it morphed into a full-time closure without warning.

At the time, John Fenik was Perth's mayor. As it happens, the mayor sits on the hospital board, which means Fenik was well aware of what the board was discussing in the lead-up to the decision to close the ER, although he had no direct authority over the hospital's operations. "When I heard that the Perth emergency department was going to close, I had discussions with the [hospital] CEO and expressed my extreme concern," Fenik said. "I asked them to do whatever needed to be done to keep the emergency department open."

Hospital authorities blamed the temporary closure on a Covid outbreak among staff at the facility. In a release, they said the outbreak had placed "yet another burden on our fragile staffing situation" and that they had "no other option" but to order the ER to close.

Dr. Al Drummond wasn't buying what the hospital was selling. "The closure was blamed on Covid, and that's totally unfair," he said. "The closure came about by virtue of experienced nurses leaving the job." It's a problem, Drummond told me, that has been years in the making. "For twenty-four years, I've been talking about the dangers of crowding and the impact in terms of staffing, safety, violence and career longevity. We've had twenty years to know about it."

What Drummond means is that even before the pandemic, Ontario was dealing with chronic problems such as a shortage of long-term care beds. That meant patients would wait weeks if not months in acute care hospitals for a space at a long-term care home to open up, and ERs like the one in Perth were constantly clogged with patients. By the time the mid-2010s rolled around, experienced nurses, despairing of their working conditions, were burning out, and few younger nurses were coming to replace them. "We had about fifteen nurses in our emergency department," Drummond explained, including full-time, part-time and casual nurses. Just before the pandemic, the ER was down to eight nurses they could count on.

The pandemic of course brought more attrition. "There were, I think, six or seven full-time staff working," Tiggy Baker said, "and it takes five staff to run the department for one shift." Then two nurses went on maternity leave, which brought the nursing complement down to five. "Of the other remaining five, two got Covid," Drummond said. "Just before the closure, we were down to three nurses. We had nurses who were working eight hours, running home, making supper for their kids and then coming back for another six or eight hours just to try and fill the gap. And we were done."

"We knew the closure was coming long before we closed," said Tiggy, disputing the idea that it came as a complete surprise to everyone involved with the hospital. "We had tried to tell management that we couldn't function. We knew it was coming. It was a matter of time." She said it upset her that the hospital made it seem as if the nurses still working were incapable of running the ER. "To have them turn around and say that it was closing because one of our colleagues got Covid was a little bit of a kick in the pants."

Drummond agreed. "It was wrong to blame it on Covid. It would have been right to say the previous administration fucked up in terms of dealing with the concerns of our nursing staff, which led us to this crisis situation. But there's no point crying over spilt milk. To be fair, I think our administration—and it was a new administration—probably did the right thing by saying that if the ED couldn't provide safe care, it probably shouldn't be providing any. The board rightly said, 'Three nurses can't do this.' And so they had to close it."

The ER in Perth was closed, but the one in Smiths Falls remained open. For veteran paramedics like Bryan Pollock, who'd worked in Lanark County for nearly thirty-three years, this added to the minute-by-minute challenge of responding to emergencies across the county's nearly 3,000 square kilometres. Each trip to Smiths Falls could add another fifteen or twenty minutes for paramedics, and when they arrived, the doctors and nurses were often overwhelmed and there were no beds. That meant crews were stuck in offload delay in the Smiths Falls ER even longer than they were before the closure in Perth. "You kind of wonder what's going to happen if that big accident occurs out on the highway and you just don't have the resources," said Pollock.

For Tiggy and the other nurses who hadn't left the ER in Perth, the closure brought chaos. "We ended up getting redeployed to the ER in Smiths Falls, which was difficult," she told me. "They definitely run a very different ER over there. It was going into an unfamiliar emergency department and working with people when you don't know how they function. I was just trying to make things work."

Meanwhile, additional Covid cases among Perth staff extended the ER closure from its original five days to a total of just over three weeks. At the same time, Al Drummond was trying to make sure that hospital administrators understood the risks that a full closure brought. "Heart attacks can occur at any time," he noted, "and so can accidents." In Perth, the ER physician on the night shift also had to respond to emergencies throughout the hospital. "If there's a cardiac arrest on a post-operative patient, who's going to look after that patient? Because there's not going to be a doctor and emergency department anymore to provide that extra level of comfort."

The hospital quickly realized that Drummond was right and backtracked enough to have an ER physician on-site in case inpatients deteriorated rapidly or someone in distress walked in off the street.

Meanwhile, others were joining the fight to reopen the emergency department. Mayor John Fenik had resigned from the hospital board immediately after the ER was closed. "I felt at the time I needed to speak on behalf of the town and the citizens of Perth," he said. "I couldn't do that when I was a board member." Once he'd left, he was free to advocate on behalf of the community. "I was making calls to the CEO of the hospital . . . I think that provided some traction. At Queen's Park, I spoke to the minister of health [and] our MPP. My message to the folks at Queen's Park started resonating."

Finally, at 7:30 a.m. on Sunday, July 24, the ER reopened.

President and CEO Michael Cohen said in a statement, "While

we all need to acknowledge that the risks posed by COVID are ever present, we have developed a strong plan to ensure that we can re-establish emergency services to our community. I want to thank the staff and physicians for all their hard work and dedication to the communities that we serve."

"I think what happened to the community was a shock," Drummond said, "because suddenly they found themselves without that guaranteed access to twenty-four seven care. A lot of people don't have the ability to drive all over God's little acre, so felt very unsettled."

Paramedic Bryan Pollock, who retired after the closure, was among those who found it unsettling. He said he felt fortunate that no one had died on his shifts because of the lack of ER access. But he wasn't prepared to say for certain that no one was harmed. After all, the ER was closed in July, when the roads and waterways were swollen with tourists, cottagers and boaters out for a good time. "When you leave work, you don't hear what goes on," he says. "I'm sure it did happen. I was lucky enough that it didn't happen with me while I was working."

Tiggy lasted another year before putting in for a transfer from the ER to the hospital's rehabilitation ward. The ER was back up and running, but the chronic shortage of nurses persisted. "You're constantly being asked to do more and more and more with less and less and less," she said. "You're expected to stay sixteen and eighteen hours . . . and then go home for maybe six hours and then come back and do a night shift."

She was doing all that while raising a family. In 2022, she says, "I did 450 hours of overtime on top of my full-time job with two kids and hockey and being a mom, and it was starting to carry over into my home life . . . I was home but I wasn't physically, emotionally and mentally present."

And it was affecting her at work as well. She felt guilty those few times when she refused a request to work overtime, but she also worried that exhaustion and sleep deprivation would lead to errors on the job. "It just got to a point where you're waking up through what little hours of sleep that you're getting," she said. "'Did I chart that? Did I sign off on that medication? Am I going to get sued for malpractice, or will somebody come back to say that I was rude or that I was not engaged?' I was not the best nurse that I know that I can be. It just got to that point where something had to change."

That a heart-and-soul nurse like Tiggy feels she has to leave a department and colleagues she loves is cause for great concern. It's an indication that the little ER in the hospital that punches above its weight may be buckling.

As Drummond said, the problems plaguing ERs across the country are decades in the making. But he surprised me by saying that he believes a repeat of Perth's ER closure is unlikely. "It was pretty concerning for the community at large and certainly for our civic politicians who put a lot of money into maintaining hospital facilities and townships. We just can't allow this to ever happen again."

Ed McPherson, the one-time paramedic and current deputy mayor, sees things a bit differently. He called closing the ER "a never event that from now [on] is all the more likely." It was like breaking a spell, he said. "Everybody is wondering, 'When is the next closure going to happen?' I think people have lost faith that the healthcare system is going to be there for them when they need it."

When I wrote *The Night Shift*, ER closures were still considered "never" events. Back then it would have taken a natural disaster like an earthquake or tsunami to force a hospital and its ER to shut its doors. Now, temporary closures are so common that they've been normalized.

Clinton, Ontario—famous as the home of a massive radar antenna that dates back to the Second World War—is a small town near the shores of Lake Huron, about a two-and-a-half-hour drive west of Toronto. Unfortunately, Clinton's hospital has had ER closures on its radar screen for longer than most other facilities. On November 9, 2019, the Huron Perth Healthcare Alliance (HPHA)—a coalition of the hospitals in Clinton, St. Marys, Seaforth and Stratford—announced that Clinton Public Hospital's ER would be closing overnights. This was supposed to be a temporary fix, but it's now going on more than four years and counting. Not only that, but the ER has had to close intermittently for full days on some weekends and civic holidays, and even occasionally on weekdays.

The shutdowns in Clinton, like the one in Perth and those at many other hospitals across Canada, are the result of an acute lack of qualified nurses—and this is nothing new. Andrew Williams, president and CEO of HPHA, told me, "In 2008, we had one of our other sites running at reduced hours in the same way we're doing [in Clinton] because of availability of nurses. There really is a challenging system issue. We don't have enough healthcare professionals for the jobs that are available."

Williams told me that there are several reasons for the chronic nursing shortage. One of the biggest, in his view, is that younger nurses yearn to specialize. "All these small rural hospitals were built at a time when healthcare professionals were generalists," he noted. "A nurse did a bit of obstetrics, a bit of emergency and a bit of internal medicine." Today's graduates, he said, want to do only one of those things. Like the medical graduate who chooses to become a specialist instead of a family doctor, young nurses are opting to specialize so they can gain mastery over a tighter scope of nursing.

A second reason is that young nurses want to be eased into the job and mentored by experienced colleagues, not thrown into the deep end of emergency medicine. This is understandable. Behind their demand for mentorship is youthful anxiety about making mistakes. "It's honestly terrifying," Holly Braecker, a young Clinton nurse, told me about working nearly alone in the ER. "A lot of days are good, but the terrifying thing is you never know when the patch [paramedic] phone will go off and what's going to come through those doors. We had a sick child a couple of weeks back who had a seizure. That's something that terrifies me. We see a lot of seniors. We don't often see younger kids."

Urban ERs may have as many as ten to fifteen nurses on duty on a given shift, but rural ERs like the one in Clinton may have only two or three nurses on duty during the day and as few as one at night. In fact, Williams told me that in Clinton they've had to increase their ER staffing to two nurses at night because people weren't comfortable working on their own. Even so, circumstances sometimes intervene. If the ER doctor orders a CT scan, for example, the patient will have to be transferred to the hospital in Stratford, which is a forty-five-minute drive away. "If we have a CT scan and a nurse has to go [with the patient], that takes away one of the nurses," Holly explained. "When we have no nurses available to come in on their day off, it leaves us in a tight situation."

Meanwhile, the ripples of those nighttime closures continue. As reported by CTV News, on July 30, 2023, a triple stabbing took place at a sweet sixteen party in Clinton. A driver took the injured teens to the hospital, less than two kilometres away, only to find the ER closed. The driver had to regroup and take them to Alexandra Marine and General Hospital in Goderich, some twenty kilometres away. One of the victims, who had a more serious puncture wound, was later airlifted to London Health Sciences Centre.

Fortunately, all three teens survived, but nevertheless the incident drew widespread reaction from the community and from authorities. "We are playing Russian roulette here," Jim Ginn, mayor of Central Huron, told the media. "Sooner or later something is going to happen here and it's going to cost someone their life. It came close this time."

Andrew Williams shares Mayor Ginn's concerns, but he has no idea how to fix things. "I don't see it getting better in the short term," he told me. In fact, he expects it to get worse because he's increasingly competing with urban hospitals for a share of the shrinking pool of nurses. "Our health system is like a round hole and our human resource supply is like a square peg. Something's got to change. We've either got to adapt the health system to the people that are out there, or we've got to adjust the education system to the needs of the health system."

What's happening in the ER in Clinton is happening at ERs across Canada.

In 2023, for example, emergency departments in Alberta were forced to close for more than 38,000 hours, or the equivalent of about 4.3 years, according to data collected by Great West Media and published by Alberta Health Services. Of the twenty-six emergency departments that shut their doors that year, more than half stayed shut for twenty days or longer.

According to Nova Scotia's *Annual Accountability Report on Emergency Departments*, that province's emergency rooms closed for 41,923 hours in the 2022–23 fiscal year, a 32 per cent year-over-year increase.

The country's most granular data on ER closures comes from Ontario—and that's because of a tenacious physician named David Savage. Savage is an ER doctor at Thunder Bay Regional Health Sciences Centre, as well as an assistant professor at the Northern Ontario School of Medicine and the site director at ICES North. ICES, the Institute for Clinical Evaluative Sciences, is a health research institute that uses such information as surveys, anonymous patient records and clinical and administrative databases to evaluate healthcare delivery and outcomes.

Savage started tracking Ontario's emergency room shutdowns after the Red Lake Margaret Cochenour Memorial Hospital closed its ER on March 26, 2022. During the closure, two patients had to be transported by ambulance to the Dryden Regional Health Centre, more than two hundred kilometres away. (The Red Lake ER reopened twenty-four hours later.)

As we've already seen, most ER shutdowns are triggered by a lack of available nurses. But the situation in Red Lake was precipitated by a lack of doctors. Dr. Akila Whiley, then chief of staff in Red Lake, told CBC News that the hospital had been dealing with a physician shortage for months before the closure. "I think we've just—we finally reached a breaking point as a group," Whiley said. "These people deserve so much better. And we all want to be able to do better, but we only have so much we can give before you're just exhausted."

Savage started thinking about the immediate impact of the closure on the people who depend on the ER. And his interest was not just a case of professional curiosity. "My wife's family is from Red Lake," he told me. "She still has family there. I was thinking [about] the challenges that her family and her parents' friends are still facing in accessing care." He noted that the Red Lake hospital is one of the most remote in the province. "I feel that northern Ontario may be disproportionately affected because of the vast geography, the lower population density and the large distances between EDs."

Soon after the shutdown in Red Lake, Savage began collecting tips on ER closures across the province. "It's not perfect tracking," he says. "I'm tracking basically through social media, mainstream media and also through hospital websites." A well-connected ER physician friend suggested he ask the Ontario Ministry of Health for data, but he decided to continue collecting it on his own, in large part so as not to be beholden to the government. "With me collecting it myself, I can do whatever I want with it. I can publish it online. I can give it to anybody."

There are 163 ERs across Ontario. In 2022, Savage documented 848 instances of an emergency department closing temporarily (which is why the number is larger than the total number of ERs across the province). In 2023, the Ontario Health Coalition, citing his data, recorded the closures of 868 emergency departments (one permanent, the remainder temporary) and 316 urgent care centres, reflecting a slow but steady year-over-year rise.

Between 2021 and 2024, of all Ontario hospitals with emergency rooms or urgent care centres, thirty-eight—or close to one in five—have experienced closures. A report by the Office of the Auditor General of Ontario found that 2024 was the province's worst year for ER closures.

Now Savage wants to take his project a step further by trying to assess the impact of ER shutdowns on patients. One of his aims is to track adverse outcomes. In the case of Red Lake, that should be doable. The Thunder Bay hospital where Savage works is a regional trauma centre and accepts patients from Red Lake. "When your ER closes and patients can't access care, the possibility of a poor outcome or something being missed, it goes up significantly," he told CTV News. In northern Ontario, he added, where the average distance between ERs can be hundreds of kilometres, "the travel burden for these patients can be quite significant." It's very possible for people to die while being transferred.

And that's not the only adverse outcome that Savage worries about. "Many rural patients go to the ED for their primary care because some communities already have a shortage of family physicians," he said. "When an ED closes, [those patients] lose both their emergency and primary care."

Savage has become a go-to source for those who write about and study healthcare issues, and his findings are quoted regularly by news organizations like the *Toronto Star* and CTV News. I ask if his project has also had an impact on the number of ER closures in Ontario.

"I'm not sure that my work has influenced much yet," he said. "[And] I have no interest in embarrassing anyone. My hope is to stimulate discussion and maybe influence policy at some point. I also enjoy research, and this seems worthwhile."

In some of Canada's smallest and most remote towns and villages, the local ER is staffed by family doctors, not emergency specialists. Overall, nursing shortfalls are the biggest problem facing the healthcare system, but in many of those small communities, the lack of doctors is the critical issue. This is what happened in Red Lake, for example, and across the country. Rural ERs are often just two or three family doctors away from having to close. Dr. Ken Milne is on a personal mission to stop that from happening.

Milne is a staff physician at the Strathroy Middlesex General Hospital in Strathroy, Ontario, just west of London, and he also teaches evidence-based medicine, clinical epidemiology, critical appraisal and biostatistics at Western University. Since 2012, he's been hosting *The Skeptics' Guide to Emergency Medicine* (The SGEM), a popular weekly podcast for doctors that aims to supercharge knowledge translation by cutting the time gap from research paper to widespread application in the ER from a decade or more to less than a year. The podcast is essential listening for family doctors who work in rural ERs in remote parts of Canada.

All of that would be a heavy workload for just about anyone, but for more than fifteen years, Milne has also been part of a variety of Ontario government programs that recruit substitute ER doctors in much the same way school boards recruit substitute teachers. "There were rural emergency departments that were really struggling," Milne told me, explaining what drew him to these programs.

"They reached out looking for physicians to help augment some of these rural places. It was an opportunity for me to learn and grow and also help out other emergency departments."

The way the program works, Milne and other MDs indicate where and how often they are willing to work as well as the dates they are available. He and others get called as soon as the word gets out that a rural Ontario ER needs a doctor for a particular shift. Milne has worked in ERs as far south as Chatham and Leamington, as far east as Pembroke and as far north as Lake of the Woods, Kenora, and Iroquois Falls. "Man, I've put a lot of kilometres on my vehicle. I think I've done close to one thousand shifts now," he told me, "preventing a thousand emergency department closures."

Milne told me one memorable story about getting a call from the provincial agency that recruits and schedules doctors like him. The person on the other end of the line said that the ER in Bancroft, Ontario, was in danger of having to close that evening for lack of MDs.

"I'd love to help you out," Milne told the person, "but I'm working a ten-hour day shift [in Strathroy] until 6 p.m." The shift in Bancroft—which was almost five hundred kilometres away—was scheduled to start at eight. There was no way he could make it.

The person from the agency asked him to reconsider.

Milne is the kind of guy who dislikes the word *impossible*. He said he'd try, and then immediately called up a fellow physician who also happened to be a pilot and asked if he could fly him to Bancroft.

Did I tell you that Ken can be extremely persuasive?

"I finish my shift. I get out to the local little airstrip. Pilot Peter picks me up in this single-engine plane. We get to Bancroft in under two hours. We had to land before sunset because the runway in Bancroft does not have lights. It's a dirt strip and a very hard place to land because there's this rolling hill in front of it. I felt a bit like Indiana Jones."

His friend managed to land the plane, and like any good Canadian, the local nurse was waiting with her pickup truck and a couple of Tim Hortons coffees. When they got to the hospital, Milne set to work while Pilot Peter went off to the doctors' sleep room so he'd be refreshed and ready to fly Milne home the next day to do a shift in Strathroy.

What strikes me about this story is that the Bancroft ER would have closed but for Milne's willingness to do the shift and a kindly friend's generosity in flying him there and back.

"That was the risk," Milne said. "There have been a lot of close calls over the years with last-minute calls. Sometimes the local physician has a family or personal emergency. Sometimes the person [who was supposed to fill in] has their own personal emergency [and] they have to go deeper into the bench. I've come in lots of times at the last minute."

Milne is far from the only physician who moonlights at rural ERs to help keep them open. But until he came along, most of the substitute ER doctors came from big cities. He was one of the first who worked at a rural ER himself. It means he has extraordinary empathy for rural physicians and understands the challenges of caring for patients in underserviced parts of the province.

Another issue Milne has to deal with is that these small ERs are habitually short-staffed. "It's just me and a couple of nurses and maybe a ward clerk helping us with documentation," he explained. "And somebody's holding up a phone to your ear so you can keep doing CPR while talking to a specialist in a larger hospital."

Multi-tasking doctors and nurses doing a lot with a little has been the norm for ages at rural and remote hospitals. But how did we go from ER closures being a never event in 2006 to being commonplace today? Milne's theory about what's behind the chronic nursing shortage is basically the same as Andrew Williams's: As medicine becomes ever more complicated, fewer and fewer people want to be generalists.

"These amazing people have slowly gone away as medicine becomes more specialized," said Milne. "It's more challenging and has become more team-based, which I fully support. But a team-based approach means you need enough team members to be there. And right now, there aren't. And since 2021, there have been a lot of ER closures" as a result.

Lately, Milne has been doing a lot of public speaking about what he calls "postal code" medicine. It's a catchy take on the notion that access to emergency medicine depends largely on where you live. "We should be practising medicine based on need. And I've always taken pride in being a Canadian and thinking that if you need care, you'll get care. And if you need emergency care, it'll be there for you. I have felt really disheartened over the last couple of years as I've seen these communities suffer with closure after closure after closure."

Along with his advocacy, Milne is working harder than ever to keep rural ERs open. "I've done more shifts in the last three years than I did when I was first out of medical school," he said. "I feel this great sense of 'What happens if I don't show up?'"

No matter when or how Milne arrives, he is greeted with smiles and sighs of relief. "It is nice to be appreciated," he told me. "I love my job and I love working with all of these wonderful nurses. The patients are fantastic and appreciative. It's nice being that person that comes in and helps. I really enjoy doing good."

But despite being an optimistic guy by nature, he's downright pessimistic about the future of rural emergency medicine. In the near term, he sees more temporary closures. Down the road, he sees more ERs closing for good. It means patients like James Keelaghan may end up with worse outcomes. It also means that people will have to travel far from their homes to ERs in larger cities to receive care. "If we close smaller places, the larger centres aren't equipped to take care of [the overflow]," he says. "They're [already] all backed up with twenty-hour waits and hallway medicine and full beds. And now, your elderly parent who has pneumonia is going to go to a big-city hospital where she doesn't know anybody, with family members far away."

Unlike Ken Milne, I work in a hospital in Canada's largest city, and I believe my ER is likely in no danger of closing. But Milne believes I have a false sense of security. He's convinced that ERs like mine are next in line to have temporary closures.

In a way, he welcomes it.

"I don't think much change will happen until [this crisis] hits suburbia."

CHAPTER SEVEN

BELIEVE

12:40 a.m.

The din in the waiting room has diminished somewhat. Three of the regulars are sleeping in chairs. In the second stretcher down the offload hallway, a slightly overweight young man with a six-inch pompadour of carrot-red hair like Conan O'Brien's is hunched over a large teal-blue plastic basin. He's retching saliva. Big, loud retches. Like a cat trying to barf up a boulder-sized hairball.

Cynthia is suddenly next to me. "Do you mind seeing Hurls?"

"I assume you mean the patient who is vomiting," I reply. "I wasn't aware he comes here often enough to earn a nickname."

"You haven't met Jimy? I thought everyone knew him. He's a young kid with cyclical vomiting who started coming here a couple of months ago."

"First time for me," I reply. "But why do you need me to see him? Isn't Samir on major?"

"He's lost somewhere in the ER maze trying to keep up," she says. "I know you're not on major, but I'm hoping you can give him something for the nausea so he can hit the road."

"I'm kind of busy myself," I start.

Cynthia gives me that "Don't frak with me" look that I envy.

I pick up the chart, grab a fresh towel (in case the patient needs it to clean off vomit) and start towards Jimy's stretcher. His heaves grow louder as I approach. We see lots of patients who come to the ER repeatedly with vomiting. Cyclical vomiting syndrome, or CVS, sounds like a made-up diagnosis, but it isn't. It's a recognized disorder that causes sudden, repeated attacks of severe nausea and vomiting. Other symptoms include abdominal pain, diarrhea, dizziness, headache and sensitivity to light. CVS often begins in children around three to seven years of age, but the number of cases diagnosed in adults is on the rise. Episodes last from a few hours to several days. In between bouts, patients may be completely fine.

Just as I arrive, Jimy retches up a bolus of spit. I don't see any yellow or green bile, which is good because it means he probably doesn't have a bowel blockage. He's sweaty and has tears in his eyes. He might be sad, but the increase in bodily fluids could be from the activation of his parasympathetic nervous system triggered by the vomiting.

"Jimy, I'm Dr. Goldman." I offer him the fresh towel.

"Thanks," he says, mopping sweat and tears off his face.

"This is your fifth visit to the ER."

"The vomiting is getting worse," he says.

"I see from your chart that you have abdominal pain and diarrhea as well." Diarrhea is not a prominent symptom of CVS. "I see that you've had lots of tests: an abdominal ultrasound, CT scan, MRI, stool cultures and lots of blood tests."

"All of them normal except low potassium and magnesium," says Jimy.

"Takes a lot of vomit for that to happen," I reply. "Your blood sugar was also on the low side."

"I've had episodes of hypoglycemia since I was a kid," he says.

"You were supposed to have an endoscopy to see if you have an ulcer," I note.

"I'm booked next month," he says.

That panel of tests is not unusual. The long list of other conditions that masquerade as CVS includes gastroenteritis, acid reflux, gallbladder disease, pancreatitis and bowel blockage. Even migraine shows up on the list because some patients with migraine have nausea but no headaches.

An increasingly common cause of recurrent vomiting and abdominal pain is cannabinoid hyperemesis syndrome, caused by heavy daily use of cannabis. Generally, patients use cannabis for several years before the onset of vomiting. Their symptoms resolve when they drastically reduce their consumption.

"How much marijuana do you use?" I ask Jimy.

"I'm not a heavy user, if that's what you're asking."

Who knows what a patient means by "heavy user" these days. If you've heard the phrase "Not your grandmother's weed," you know what I mean. When doctors talk about the potency of cannabis, they're referring to the percentage of tetrahydrocannabinol, or THC, the key psychoactive ingredient in the product. It causes euphoria, sedation, drowsiness—and vomiting. According to Health Canada, the strength of the cannabis available back in the 1980s was 3 per cent THC give or take. Today, it's routinely around 15 per cent, and can be a lot higher.

Jimy's not making eye contact with me. Mostly he looks like he's trying to tough out his illness. But at just eighteen, he still has one foot in childhood.

"Nice tat," I tell him. He has a turntable and a set of headphones sleeve-tattooed to his left shoulder. "Are you a DJ?"

"Giving it a shot," he says.

"Tell me about your family."

"Not much to tell," he replies. "They don't approve of my career choice. I was an art major before I flunked out of first year."

The diagnostic wheels are starting to turn in my head. There are lots of possibilities.

Could Jimy have an eating disorder? The National Eating Disorders Association in the US says roughly one in three people struggling with an eating disorder is male. Because of cultural and gender bias, males are much less likely than women to be assessed or diagnosed for their eating disorder, and even less likely to seek treatment.

"Are you trying to lose weight?" I ask him.

"Who isn't?"

I turn on the flashlight on my phone. "Let me take a quick look inside your mouth," I say.

There are no mouth sores, which we see in patients with bulimia. Jimy's teeth also look okay. There's no erosion of the surface enamel from chronic vomiting.

"What's that?" I notice a callus on Jimy's index finger, where it meets the palm. Injuries to the digits are often seen in patients who induce vomiting by sticking their fingers down their throat.

"I told you, I'm a DJ," says Jimy shortly. "It's from flicking discs."

"Sorry, I forgot." I'm alienating my patient and not getting closer to the diagnosis. I decide to treat his nausea and come back when I have more information. "Let's get some blood work. We'll give you some IV fluids and ondansetron to treat the nausea."

"Do you mind giving me dimenhydrinate instead of ondansetron?" he asks. "I find it works better."

"You know what works," I reply. "Let's see how you are in a while."

At the triage station I write up the chart and tell Cynthia the plan. "In addition to the blood work, can you get an ECG?" I ask. "Can you also get a urine toxicology screen? I want to see if he's still using cannabis."

"Doesn't everybody who shows up here?" she asks rhetorically.

I don't like vomiting as a symptom because I can't discharge

Jimy until he demonstrates at minimum that he can drink fluids without throwing up. I also don't like not knowing why my patient is vomiting. I'm pretty sure there's something Jimy isn't telling me.

As a medical student, I was taught that the most effective way to make a diagnosis is to listen to what a patient tells you. Once out in practice, you learn that patients also sometimes conceal information. Knowing when to believe the patient and when to call BS is one of the greatest challenges of clinical practice.

Jimy is not the first patient I've seen who I believe is being selective in what he tells me. Like every ER physician, I've seen lots of patients who withhold pertinent facts.

Dr. Gregory House was once TV's most popular physician. His motto, "Everybody lies," was the operating principle that he used to make rare and unusual diagnoses. House's credo is the corollary of an enduring principle known as Occam's razor, which holds that if you have competing explanations for a situation, phenomenon or diagnosis, the simplest one is usually the correct one.

Once you know whether a patient is concealing the truth, it's a lot easier to figure out which of the explanations is the simplest.

Patients often conceal details about their dietary, sexual or other habits because they fear things like legal consequences, shame and stigma. "Many patients lie or withhold medically important information from their doctors," wrote journalist Lauren Vogel in a 2019 issue of *CMAJ*, the journal of the Canadian Medical Association. She cited two American studies in which 60 to 80 per cent of those surveyed said they had not been forthcoming with their physicians about information that could have been relevant to their health and well-being. Nearly half acknowledged that they had lied to their doctors about their diets and exercise routines, their sexual habits and practices or their compliance with doctor-recommended treatments.

Some patients lie because they fear their doctors will confront them about their habits and behaviours or judge them harshly. There's some evidence to suggest that their fears are justified. A 2016 survey of doctors published in *Medscape*, a news and education resource for health professionals, found that 40 per cent of physicians in the US hold biases towards patients who are obese, have emotional problems or have difficulty speaking and understanding English. Among American ER physicians, the number rose to a whopping 62 per cent.

When I was a much younger ER physician, I published articles and gave lots of lectures and workshops on how to recognize people who pretend to have illnesses to obtain prescriptions for opioid pain relievers. Before the arrival of cheap and plentiful fentanyl, scamming doctors was one of the more productive ways to obtain opioids for recreational use.

I used to delight in having what I thought of as an intrinsic "lie detector." I would ask patients if they had obtained prescriptions from other physicians, and if so, to give me the date of the most recent prescription. If they said they hadn't received any prescriptions lately, I would confirm their account with colleagues and nearby pharmacies. I especially enjoyed it when the extra effort and time spent obtaining that collateral information helped me catch patients in a fib.

Decades of emergency medicine made me very confident in judging when to believe patients and when to disbelieve them. It also gave me that extra shot of courage that enabled me to play the role of "truth teller"—confronting lies where I detected them and helping patients see and receive the truths they did not wish to know.

Around a decade ago, I saw a young married woman who was

physically assaulted by her then husband on a highly significant day in their social calendar. Her injuries were minor and easily treated, fortunately. I vividly recall taking her to a quiet place in the ER and telling her that the natural history of domestic violence tilts like magnetic north towards more frequent and more dangerous acts of violence.

"Things will only get worse for you," I recall telling her in no uncertain terms. "You must leave this relationship now."

Like most spouses who experience intimate partner violence, she appeared traumatized. She also looked stunned that I had recommended she terminate a fundamental relationship in which she was fully invested.

We said goodbye and I went to see the next patient. Who knew what she would do with my forceful act of telling it like it was.

A few years later, on a busy ER shift, I was summoned to the triage area. My first thought was that I was being called to try to placate a patient who was dissatisfied with some aspect of my care. But I was wrong.

It was her. Her hair looked different, but it was definitely her.

She hadn't expected to see me. She said she had just wanted to drop off a note to tell me what had happened. When the admitting clerk realized I was on duty, she summoned me.

The woman's note said it all. She took in what I had said, packed a bag and left her husband that very night. She started fresh, went back to school and was living a new life.

I was the truth teller who said things that likely tracked with what she was already thinking and feeling. Perhaps I helped shatter her belief in the illusion of a mostly happy and successful relationship.

If I hadn't confronted her and challenged her beliefs, she might have stayed in the marriage longer—perhaps too long. Or she might have left the marriage that night all on her own.

When you receive feedback like that, you can't help but think that you know exactly when to believe patients and when to call them on their fibs and self-deceptions. That you recognize the space where believing the patient ends and skepticism begins.

Late in my career, a most unusual patient taught me a huge lesson about that.

You may have heard about this patient because she was the subject of a 2024 case report published in *CMAJ* by Dr. Rahel Zewude, a specialist in infectious diseases, and several of her colleagues. The article documents her incredible story and became a news sensation in Canada and around the world.

The patient was a fifty-year-old woman who went to the ER with symptoms of alcohol intoxication. Not once or twice but seven times over a two-year period. On the seventh visit, the patient's story took a detour that changed both the narrative and her life. I know that because I'm the ER physician who saw her on that seventh occasion, a night shift. (Dr. Zewude acknowledged this in her *CMAJ* paper by asking me to be one of the paper's co-authors.)

One day nearly three years earlier, the woman (who asked not to be named) started having episodes of inexplicable daytime sleepiness and what she described as "weakness." For instance, she would fall asleep suddenly while getting ready for work or preparing meals. She went to see her family doctor, who had no explanation for her symptoms.

The woman believed her sleepiness might be connected to foods she was eating. She tried fasting and soon noticed a pattern: "I stop eating, then I feel better." For two or three days, she would limit herself to water or tea without milk. She also tried an ancient

Ayurvedic remedy called Triphala, which is a blend of three fruits. The remedy is believed to detoxify, cleanse and support digestion. It may help reduce inflammation and protect against some cancers. It may also help with constipation, dental issues and weight loss. After several days of fasting and taking Triphala, the woman always felt better. Until the cycle would repeat itself.

Over time, her symptoms began to affect her work. She had to take time off whenever she got sick. Her co-workers noticed she wasn't well. "They know me from the last thirty years," she explained to me in an interview. "They saw me growing there, saw me giving birth to kids. The entire crew knows me. They used to tell me, 'You're going to get help.'"

As the episodes became more frequent, she took a leave of absence, which triggered a family crisis. "It's not only me alone. It's my whole entire family with me," she said. "I'm not going to work. I have to pay [the] mortgage. I'm lying in a bed. I'm looking for help. It was very painful."

This is when she started frequenting ERs. Her visits were triggered by falls, but the doctors noticed something else: slurred speech and the smell of alcohol on her breath.

With findings like these, most ER physicians I know will suspect the patient is intoxicated with booze. The way to confirm the diagnosis is to obtain a blood alcohol concentration, or BAC for short, to detect alcohol in the bloodstream. We order a BAC if the patient is in a coma and there is serious doubt about the cause, if we suspect the patient is using alcohol in combination with an opioid like fentanyl or if there are other potential causes of stupor, such as a head injury. We also order a BAC if a patient is at risk of developing acute alcohol withdrawal, which can be life-threatening.

As documented in the case report in *CMAJ*, doctors diagnosed acute alcohol intoxication on the woman's first six visits to the ER. On some of those occasions, they confirmed the diagnosis with a BAC. At every visit, they told the patient that she had been drinking.

"In the past, she would drink a glass of wine on holidays; however, in recent years, she had stopped drinking altogether because of her religious beliefs," Zewude wrote.

On three of her visits to the ER, the doctors who saw her were so convinced she had an alcohol problem that they referred her to a psychiatrist to help her deal with it. On the third of those three visits, the woman tried to leave the ER, prompting the physician to "certify" her under provincial mental health legislation. That meant she couldn't leave the hospital voluntarily and had to submit to a mandatory psychiatric assessment.

In describing this bizarre and seemingly unsolvable situation to me, the woman talked about feeling despair, but her voice and her demeanour were serene. "What can I do?" she asked. "I cried a lot. But at home, I had such a strong help from my husband and my sister and my own child, who were telling me, 'We believe.'"

On my shift in the ER, the patient arrived with slurred speech and the odour of alcohol on her breath, as she had on the six previous visits. When I asked her how much alcohol she drinks, as before she insisted that she did not consume any whatsoever.

My first thought was that she was in denial, which is a key symptom of problem drinking. I planned to confront her about her alcohol use, but it was a busy night shift, and I decided to put off the conversation until I had the results of her BAC. Some ER physicians would have skipped the blood test and confronted her then and there. Looking back, I wonder if I was stalling. I've always felt uncomfortable confronting patients about drug and alcohol use and other unhealthy habits because they often get angry and push back. I've improved with age, but I still have trouble dealing with that.

There are compelling reasons for ER physicians to get better at challenging patients about their drinking. Alcohol consumption is a proven public health problem. For instance, the Canadian Cancer Society says having three to four drinks a day raises the risk of breast and colorectal cancer by 50 per cent and doubles the risk of cancer of the mouth, throat, larynx and esophagus. A 2018 study of 195 countries, published in the journal *The Lancet*, found that alcohol was the leading risk factor for death among people ages fifteen to forty-nine.

The ER is typically the entry point to the healthcare system for patients with alcohol-related health problems. It's not surprising, then, that ER physicians are being encouraged to identify unhealthy drinking habits not just in those whose issues are obvious but in every patient they see.

The alcohol level on my patient came back at 62 millimoles per litre. A normal blood alcohol level is less than 2 millimoles per litre, so I now had proof that the patient was intoxicated. In my clinical experience, the only explanation was that she'd been drinking. For the good of her health, the advocate in me said I had to confront her. But when I did, she once again insisted that she didn't drink.

This was when her friend who accompanied her to the ER pulled me aside and told me that she had stopped drinking alcohol for religious reasons. She asked me if the patient could be suffering from a condition she had read about on the internet called alcohol auto-intoxication syndrome.

I had heard of the condition but had never had occasion to diagnose it myself. I said I'd look it up. What I found was that it's more commonly called auto-brewery syndrome. It's an extremely rare condition—only a few dozen cases have been reported in medical journals since the syndrome was first described in Japan in 1952—but it is a recognized disease in which a person's body makes its own alcohol by fermenting dietary carbs in the gastrointestinal tract. In other words, you don't have to drink alcohol to get drunk. The body does it for you.

As I read more, I learned that this condition develops when a patient's gut gets colonized by fermenting fungi such as *Saccharomyces cerevisiae* and *Candida albicans* or by a bacterium named *Klebsiella pneumoniae*.

I asked my patient where her friend got the notion that she had auto-brewery syndrome.

"My family is very inquisitive by nature," she told me. "One of them asked for help in the university where she was studying, and then she did research and she talked to my friend."

Her friend also had help from other family members, some of whom were doctors and engineers. "They said, 'Go tell your doctor and ask them if they can do tests [for auto-brewery syndrome],'" the patient explained. "My friend just communicated that these are the thoughts given to us. 'Can we try that one to get it checked?' That is how it came to you."

"Son of a gun," I thought. Here was a plausible explanation for the patient's alcohol intoxication.

My mind started to shift. I asked myself why the woman had returned to the ER yet again. If she was in denial about an alcohol problem, she would have had no incentive to see yet another ER physician and be diagnosed once again with alcohol use disorder. The best explanation was that she came back hoping that someone would view her symptoms with a fresh set of eyes. I've seen hundreds if not thousands of patients over the decades who return to the ER in search of a diagnosis for an unsolved medical problem. Why not her?

Thanks to a big assist from her friend and from her family, I decided to believe her. The treatment guidelines I'd read online recommended a prescription for fluconazole, an antimicrobial that kills fungi. By the way, antibiotics specifically target bacteria, while antimicrobials are a broader category that includes drugs effective against a wider range of microbes, including bacteria, viruses, fungi and parasites. Since auto-brewery syndrome is caused by a fungal infection, this treatment made sense. So I prescribed fluconazole, and then I referred her to a gastroenterologist instead of a psychiatrist.

As luck would have it, my referral landed in the inbox of Dr. Ken Croitoru, a veteran GI specialist. Croitoru had done research on the gut microbiome—the fungi, bacteria and other germs that live in the digestive tract—and the role those germs play in bowel diseases.

"Something about the referral really intrigued me," Croitoru told me in an interview. "I thought this would be a patient who obviously has some altered microbiome that makes her susceptible to auto-brewery syndrome."

Many gastroenterologists might have been perplexed by the condition, in part because it's so rare. Croitoru was so taken with the referral that he saw my patient a week later. By the time he saw her, the fluconazole was having an effect, and my patient was having fewer episodes of intoxication. "I had no reason not to believe her," said Croitoru. "You gave her a prescription for fluconazole. You also told her to change her diet, and she already had a partial response to that. It wasn't an issue as to whether or not she was a closet alcoholic. To me, it was a question of how are we going to treat this definitively."

Croitoru and Dr. Ronit Das referred her to Dr. Bryan Coburn and Dr. Isaac Bogoch, both specialists in infectious diseases, and Dr. Zewude, who at the time had finished her residency in infectious diseases and was doing some post-residency training. All of them including me were co-authors of the paper in *CMAJ*. A battery of tests eventually confirmed the diagnosis. But there were still hiccups, most notably that the patient continued to have frequent bouts of alcohol intoxication. She was put on a low-carb diet to reduce the amount of fermentation—and therefore the amount of alcohol production—in her gut. The woman told me the diet was the hardest part to get right. "First they cut everything . . . They would not allow me any grain. They wouldn't allow me flour. I still don't eat wheat. I don't eat pasta . . . I do not eat [foods] from outside [the home]."

Fluconazole and a stringent diet put the brewery in her gut at bay and gave her a four-month reprieve. But when she relaxed her diet, her problems recurred. So her GI doctors gave her another two weeks of fluconazole and put her back on the low-carb diet. This time, the treatment worked. Six months later, they gave her a test dose of 150 grams of oral glucose, which is a huge hit of carbs, to see if her gut was still capable of making alcohol. Over the next forty-eight hours, they measured her blood alcohol level eight times. The upshot? No detectable alcohol in her bloodstream. None. Nada.

My patient isn't cured. She still has occasional episodes of auto-intoxication. But when she does, she reverts to the low-carb diet and her symptoms quickly clear. And she hasn't been back to the ER since the night we met.

After all she went through, I was surprised but heartened to hear that she bore no ill will towards the doctors who were convinced she was drinking. But she also made a point of telling me that she was sustained by the support of her family. "I would strongly say if my husband, my family, my sister, my brother [weren't] there, it would have been so hard for me. Maybe I would be shattered because of that. I picture other people. I don't know how they would deal with it."

This life-altering episode reinforced her empathy. "People should never give up," she told me. "If they think other people cannot understand them, they have to put themselves in their shoes." It's possible, she said, that she would have done exactly what those first six doctors did. But she also had faith that someone would eventually listen to her story. "As long as [people are] honest, they will be heard," she said. "Doctors can help [us] only when we help them [by] giving the full information. Tell them everything and don't give up."

By sending my patient to a specialist, I got the ball rolling on her formal diagnosis of auto-brewery syndrome. The spark, however, came not from me but from family members who stayed curious and not judgmental, and were driven to the correct destination by a successful trip through the internet.

This is far from the only time that Dr. Google turned out to be right.

The summer of 2024 marked a huge milestone in the life of Ian Stedman. It was the tenth anniversary of Ian's being able to go to the beach on a summer's day wearing shorts and a T-shirt instead of hiding his rash-covered skin. It was also ten years since he and his daughter Lia were diagnosed with a genetic disorder caused by a mutation in the CIAS1 / NLRP3 gene.

For more than three decades, Ian had lived with an unidentified debilitating condition and no treatment. He likely had his first symptoms as an infant. "The earliest thing I can remember would probably be arthritis or joints that weren't working properly," he told me. He also had hives, fevers, pounding headaches and a bright red rash that covered his entire body. His eyes were bloodshot. Random joints—a knuckle, a knee—flared up with arthritis. "The worst was when it was a heel or an ankle, because then you just couldn't get around. You can't go to school and you can't play. You can't do anything."

By the time he turned eighteen, he'd seen 180 doctors—numerous family doctors and many specialists, including dermatologists, rheumatologists and ophthalmologists. Each one ran some tests but sent him away without a diagnosis. Finally, he stopped searching for answers. As an adult, he learned to live with his symptoms even though he often missed days or even weeks of law school and later work as a lawyer. "I've had to be accommodated by my employers my whole life, every single job I can think of," he explained on an episode of *White Coat, Black Art*. "As a practising lawyer, I had people coming in to meet me where I've been unable to take that appointment. Those are the moments where you think, 'This is a career-limiting issue.'"

By the time Ian met and married his wife, Aimy, he had completely given up on a diagnosis. That changed in a hurry after their first daughter, Lia, was born in 2012.

"In her first year of life, the . . . rash started appearing, the one that looked like mine and looked like the one my mother had," he said. "It started appearing to the point where it was blatantly, patently obvious to everyone who saw that it was the same thing."

For Lia's sake, Ian was determined to take another crack at solving the mystery. Only this time, he wasn't a debilitated child himself but a lawyer with an analytical mind. And he was armed with two undeniable truths: First, that he and Lia both had the same symptoms meant their condition must be genetic, and second, that no doctor could identify it meant it must be rare. This is when he turned to Dr. Google . . . sort of.

"You get to the end of the rope," he recalled. "You have no idea what's next and you're just throwing everything at the wall to see what sticks. You're looking everywhere to try to figure out what you're supposed to be looking for." In desperation, he started searching online for photos of rashes that looked like his. But to be clear, this was a far more focused and curated search than simply googling the word "*rash.*" Instead, he turned to the website RareConnect, an international patient organization where people with rare diseases could connect with others. (RareConnect was retired in 2023, but posts and comments can still be accessed online.)

He looked at "thousands of photos" and read "a few dozen different stories" posted by patients, just hoping to find something that would shed light on his and Lia's situation. One night in 2013, Ian hit pay dirt. "I saw my skin," he told me, describing a moment he will never forget. "The person who had [posted the photos] described these other symptoms. I had never pieced together all these other things . . . the red eyes, the headaches, the fevers, the arthritis. Like it was my skin. It was my issue. That was what I was looking for." The website identified the person's condition as Muckle-Wells syndrome, or MWS.

Ian took a day or two to digest what he had found. But he believed he finally had a name for a disease he had been living with for thirty-two years. Now he needed a physician to validate his suspicion. Once again, an online search took him an important step forward. He discovered a conference of experts in rare diseases, including MWS. One of them was Dr. Ronald Laxer, a pediatric rheumatologist at SickKids and an internationally recognized expert in MWS and related diseases.

Armed with Laxer's email address, Ian sent him a message late at night. It landed on Laxer's phone just as he was waking up in Denmark, where he was to give a talk on MWS at a meeting of rheumatologists. "I was really intrigued," the doctor said. "It's a rare disease, but I [thought] he might be right." He emailed back suggesting that he and Ian arrange for a consultation.

As soon as Laxer got back from Denmark, the two men met and the doctor set up some special genetic testing. In early 2014, that testing finally confirmed the diagnosis of MWS. To say the condition is rare is an understatement. MWS is so uncommon that to date just sixty Canadians have ever been diagnosed with it. Ian and Lia were the eleventh and twelfth patients identified. Ian's mother was patient number thirteen.

But even though Muckle-Wells syndrome is ultra-rare, there is an effective treatment for it: a medication called canakinumab, what doctors call a "biologic" medicine (meaning it comes from living organisms).

"We started treatment and every one of our painful symptoms disappeared immediately," wrote Ian in 2016 in a blog posted on the SickKids website. "Having treatment also means that Lia will not develop long-term damage such as hearing loss in the future, something that I unfortunately already have." The treatment also prevents the organ damage that once meant that one in three people with MWS did not live to age thirty-five. But it comes at quite a cost: around $100,000 a year. Horribly expensive, but worth every penny.

I first met the Stedman clan in 2016, when Ian was thirty-four and Lia was four. Now, eight years on, they're living normal, healthy lives. "We've never had any relapses and never had any dose changes," Ian told me. He has since learned how to give himself and Lia shots of the medication every eight weeks.

And Ian's personal search for a rare diagnosis has led to an equally rare and meteoric career path. He is now an associate professor of Canadian public law and governance in the School of Public Policy and Administration at York University and is cross-appointed to graduate programs in science and technology studies and socio-legal studies at Osgoode Hall Law School. Ian also advocates for the rare disease community, and in 2025, he became the chair of the advisory board for the Institute of Genetics at the Canadian Institutes of Health Research, the first social scientist to hold that office.

Ian wants to help doctors make more one-in-a-million diagnoses by giving them tools like artificial intelligence and by opening their minds. Dr. Google helped Ian self-diagnose his rare disease, just as Dr. Google helped the family member of my intoxicated patient land on auto-brewery syndrome. Ian said, "I think we'd be crazy to expect people who are sick to not look up their symptoms and to try to figure out what they might have and whether there's anything they can do to stay out of the doctor's office!"

Had I not been prompted by the patient's friend, I doubt I would have made the auto-brewery diagnosis. Had Ian come to my ER complaining of skin rash, bloodshot eyes and painful joints, I doubt I'd have come up with MWS in a million years.

It's one thing not to recognize a plausible diagnosis because it's rare. It's something else to disbelieve the suggested diagnosis simply because it comes from the patient.

I told Ian the story of my patient with auto-brewery syndrome and how she'd been in the ER six times before she got any relief. "The first thing that struck me was how it must feel to go to doctor after doctor and have nobody believe you," he said. "I know it's not uncommon for patients to encounter disbelief when they have rare conditions, but in this case the disbelief was not about their symptoms but about what caused them. To feel like you are being accused of drinking alcohol when your religion actually prohibits you from doing so must feel doubly insulting!"

Ian said he too encountered skepticism as he closed in on the self-diagnosis of MWS. Before he could even see Dr. Ron Laxer, the pediatric rheumatologist, he had to get a referral letter from the most recent specialist who had seen him (and had failed to make a diagnosis). "I was told by the specialist, 'There's no way you have that disease! Most people with that disease are very sick, and you don't seem to be.'"

I asked him if his story represented the triumph of Dr. Google, but he was more hesitant than I expected.

"It is and it isn't," he said. "While I can appreciate that I might not have found my answers without using Google image search, I often reflect on how long it took me and how hard it was for me to get to the point where I felt smart enough to try to find my own answers. I was in a very privileged and very educated position before I ever felt confident or bold enough to try to find answers for myself."

So he recognizes that not everyone will get a successful diagnosis from digging around online, but he agrees that it was triumphant in my patient's case and his. "I might not be here today if it wasn't for my ability to search the internet and look at images of rashes from all over the world for hours on end to try to find one that looked like my own."

And there may be more diagnostic triumphs on the internet in the years to come, thanks to artificial intelligence. Recently, Ian saw AI's potential up close.

A while back, Michael Brudno, a professor in the Department of Computer Science at the University of Toronto and the chief data scientist at the University Health Network, asked Ian if he could try using AI to diagnose him faster. Brudno took all of Ian's health records, digitized them and ran them through his machine learning algorithm to see how fast it could come up with a list of plausible diagnoses for Ian's symptoms. "He had me differentially diagnosed by visit number eight with one of two autoinflammatory diseases, one being Muckle-Wells syndrome," Ian remarked.

Eight visits to the doctor instead of a hundred and eighty over thirty-two years!

It makes me wonder just how much better patients could get at self-diagnosis if they had AI at their fingertips. "I absolutely believe that artificial intelligence will be what drives the future of rare disease diagnosis, care and treatment," Ian told me. He believes that AI will bring advancements that change the practice of medicine, and that those benefits could accrue to patients online.

"The idea that we might be able to make AI-based tools available to patients who are looking for answers isn't far-fetched," he said. "They already have easy access to tools like ChatGPT and other large language models. The real question is how we make sure these tools are safe and accurate, especially if we accept that they will be used by patients who are looking for answers. I think this is an area where we still need to do some work. If we are thoughtful and careful about regulating what search tools are available online and how they can be accessed for the purpose of diagnostic advice, then perhaps we can get to a place where patients are using these tools and coming to their doctors with a differential diagnosis already in hand and ready for discussion."

1:20 a.m.

I'm thinking of my patient with auto-brewery syndrome and of Ian Stedman as I click on Jimy's electronic chart at a workstation. His serum sodium and potassium levels are below the normal range but not dangerously so. Both can be explained by his protracted vomiting. His blood alcohol level is less than 2 millimoles per litre, which means I can scratch nausea caused by alcohol intoxication from the list. More important, his urine toxicology screen is negative for THC, which means his vomiting isn't the result of cannabis use. That removes an important diagnostic possibility about which I was quite suspicious.

I still think he's not being completely candid with me. But how can I get him to open up?

My first impression as I approach his stretcher is that the antinausea medication I gave him is doing the trick. He's no longer sweaty. I resolve to be less confrontational with him.

"How are you feeling, Jimy?" I ask.

"Better, thanks."

"I've got your test results," I tell him. "They show that you were a bit dehydrated when you were brought in, but we fixed that. And," I quickly add, "your urine tested negative for cannabis."

"I told you I stopped using a few weeks ago," he says.

"You did indeed," I reply. "Sorry if I came across as pushy before. I know it's unpleasant to be vomiting, and especially to be vomiting in a hallway in the ER. I just want you to know I'm on your side. I'm puzzled by one thing, though. Cyclical vomiting, which is the name of the medical condition that causes bouts of vomiting, usually begins in childhood. Your vomiting started recently. That suggests some new factor. Do you have any additional information—even a tiny clue—that can help me figure this out?"

The look on Jimy's face changes just slightly.

"You were right when you first saw me," he says finally. "I was trying to lose weight. I bought Ozempic online."

There's the missing link! Ozempic is the trade name of semaglutide, an anti-diabetic medication that's known for causing nausea and vomiting, especially when patients just start taking it. Semaglutide treats type 2 diabetes by getting the pancreas to produce more insulin and stopping the liver from releasing too much sugar into the bloodstream. But what has turned it into a social phenomenon is that it helps people lose weight by making them feel full sooner and by stimulating the part of the brain that regulates hunger.

Semaglutide is approved in Canada for weight loss in patients diagnosed with obesity. The drug is also approved for patients who are significantly overweight and have at least one related medical condition, such as high blood pressure, type 2 diabetes or obstructive sleep apnea.

But a lot of people have taken these medications for uses that aren't medically approved. I first became acquainted with that a couple of years ago, when I had a patient in the ER with severe vomiting. Unlike Jimy, this patient told me straight up that she'd got hold of a prescription for Ozempic and was taking it because she was getting married in a month and wanted to lose five kilograms so she could fit into her wedding dress.

"How much did you inject?" I ask Jimy.

He pulls up his T-shirt. I count four small puncture wounds.

"You didn't inject all of them at once!"

"I took one the first two times," says Jimy. "When I wasn't losing weight fast enough, I took two."

The manufacturer says a higher starting dose increases the risk of side effects like nausea, vomiting and low blood sugar. Other potentially serious side effects include pancreatitis, gallbladder problems, changes in vision, kidney problems and thyroid cancer. Assuming what Jimy bought was actually semaglutide, the dose itself explains the way he's been feeling.

Diagnosing Jimy is one thing. Where we go from here is another thing altogether.

"Anytime you take something that wasn't prescribed to you, there's a risk of harm," I say. "That's why you always have to take medication under your doctor's supervision."

"Am I going to be okay?" Jimy asks. He has a concerned look on his face.

"You should be fine once the drug has worked its way out of your system. Maybe there's a lesson here."

Since Jimy is able to keep down fluids, it's safe to discharge him. I give him a few more doses of dimenhydrinate to get him through the next couple of hours and send him on his way. I'm hopeful we've seen the last of Hurls, but I have my doubts. I may have averted a crisis, but the bigger issue is why Jimy is determined to go to such lengths to lose weight when he isn't all that heavy. If he has an underlying eating disorder, I'm not going to diagnose it tonight.

Jimy and my patient with auto-brewery syndrome are at two ends of a continuum. In the mind of an ER physician, faith and doubt co-exist. The woman whose gut fermented alcohol tells me that some patients should be believed. But Jimy reminds me that it's sometimes life-saving to be skeptical. The uneasy art of emergency medicine is figuring out which patients fall into which group.

CHAPTER EIGHT

BAD THINGS HAPPEN TO YOUNG PATIENTS TOO

1:40 a.m.

Ahu approaches me with a concerned look on her face. She could have called me. That she didn't tells me she has news to deliver and wants to see my reaction when she does it.

"What's up?" I ask her.

"I just spoke to the radiology resident about Britany's CT scan," she says. Britany is the double-jointed woman who came in with severe abdominal pain. Ahu presented her to me a couple of hours ago. "She has an aortic dissection."

"Let's take a look at her CT," I suggest as we find an unoccupied computer terminal.

Ahu clicks on the transverse views, which allow us to look at a cross-section of Britany's chest. As the images come up, her eyes widen noticeably.

"Yikes!" she says, pointing to a 5.3 centimetre irregular blob of white CT contrast material.

"The ascending aorta is enlarged, all right," I tell her. My eyes dart through the images until I find a faint black diagonal line transecting the white blob. "That's the rip in the inner lining of her aorta. How do we classify dissections?"

"There are two classification systems," says Ahu. "The one I'm most familiar with is called the Stanford classification. It divides dissections into type A and type B. Type A involves the ascending aorta, and type B the descending aorta. As emergency physicians, the most important thing for us to figure out is whether Britany needs surgery."

"What about the other classification?"

"It's called the DeBakey classification, and it has three types depending on where the dissection originates," she says. "Type I involves the ascending aorta, aortic arch and descending aorta, type II is the ascending aorta, and type III is confined to the descending aorta distal to the left subclavian artery."

"Why is that classification important?"

"It matters to cardiovascular surgeons because it helps them figure out the long-term outcome from the surgical approach. It can also indicate how often they'll need to go back in and do more surgery."

"You sound like a surgeon," I reply with a note of curiosity.

"It's not that," she says. "My grandfather died suddenly on his seventy-eighth birthday from an aortic dissection. It was pretty shocking. He passed out and died right in front of us."

"I'm sorry about that."

"Thanks." Ahu looks away from me. "I thought of going into surgery, but then I did my ER rotation and changed my mind."

"So what's the bottom line, Ahu?"

"Since Britany's dissection is in the ascending aorta, it means she has a type A dissection. And that means she needs surgery to repair it."

"What about type B dissections?"

"Type B dissections are managed with medications to control blood pressure."

"Let's go tell Britany about her CT," I tell Ahu. "Would you like to give her the news?"

"You bet," she says.

In less than a minute, we arrive at Britany's stretcher in the hallway.

"How's your pain?" Ahu asks.

"It's better since I got the hydromorphone shot."

"We got the CT results," I tell her. "Ahu's going to explain because she knows way more about it than I do."

Ahu swallows hard as she glances at me. I nod to her, hoping that she sees the gesture as the vote of confidence it is.

"Britany, you have what we call an aortic dissection." Ahu gathers herself before she carries on. "It means you have a tear in your aorta, which is the big artery that comes off the heart. The aorta curves up towards your neck before curving back down into the middle of your chest and then into your abdomen. The good news is that the tear is small and confined to the uppermost part of the aorta inside the chest, called the aortic arch. That's good news because it means you're a candidate to have it repaired surgically."

"Maybe I'm too doped up on hydromorphone to be as scared as I should be," says Britany. "I'm just glad that you found the cause, and that it's fixable. But why did you ask me earlier if I'm double-jointed?"

"We were wondering about your ligaments. We use the word *double-jointed*, but that's a misnomer," Ahu explains. "What's really happening is that the ligaments around your joints are so lax that, in your case, you can bend your thumb so it's touching your wrist. We know that the inner layer of your aorta is made of the same kind of connective tissue as your ligaments. Because your ligaments are lax, that tells us that your aorta is prone to getting torn away from the surrounding layers."

Britany starts to cry. "Why did this happen to me?"

"We don't know for sure," I tell her, "but we think you were born with a genetic condition called Ehlers-Danlos syndrome. That's what makes your body's connective tissue weaker than it should be."

"Why didn't I know about it until now?"

"I'm not sure," I tell her. "There are many variations of Ehlers-Danlos, and you don't have some of the more obvious visible features, such as stretchy skin or fragile skin. Maybe that's why it was missed."

"Well, I'm happy you found it," says Britany.

"So are we," I tell her. "I've missed the diagnosis before. But as Ahu said, the important thing is that the cardiovascular surgeons should be able to fix it. That's our next step."

Ahu and I leave Britany to process everything we've just told her and head down the hallway.

"We don't have a cardiovascular surgeon here," Ahu says as we take another look at the scan. "I'll contact CritiCall. Hopefully they'll be able to find us a surgeon with hospital beds to spare." CritiCall Ontario is a provincial agency that triages patients and allocates specialists and hospital beds based on availability and urgency.

"What should we do in the meantime?" I ask.

"We need to monitor Britany's blood pressure to reduce the strain on her aorta," she says. "We should also move her to the resuscitation room in case she crashes."

I nod my agreement. "You handled that discussion really well."

"Thanks," Ahu replies. "She's so young. Not like my grandfather."

"As a mentor told me many years ago, bad things happen to young patients too."

That bad things sometimes happen to young patients has been a running theme throughout my long career as an ER physician. It's a random thing I've seen again and again.

When I was doing a night shift a few years ago, paramedics

brought in a twenty-two-year-old man in full cardiac arrest. He'd been at a gym, exercising on an elliptical trainer, when he passed out and fell to the floor. The night manager heard the thud and found the patient. She called 911, pulled the automatic external defibrillator off its wall mount and attached the adhesive electrodes on the patient. The AED detected a shockable rhythm, and the manager shocked the young man twice, with no response. She then started cardiopulmonary resuscitation and continued doing that until paramedics arrived.

The paramedics took over CPR, intubated the man, applied oxygen and started an IV. When they put the patient on a cardiac monitor, they found that he was in ventricular fibrillation, a shockable rhythm. They shocked the patient four more times. On the fourth shock, they got the patient back into a normal rhythm. Despite that, he had no recordable blood pressure, which meant his heart muscle was no longer functioning. En route to the hospital, paramedics gave the patient several doses of epinephrine to try to get the heart pumping again. To no avail.

By the time the paramedics arrived at my ER, the young man had been in cardiac arrest with no recordable blood pressure for over forty minutes. They moved him onto a stretcher in the resuscitation room, and five nurses, a respiratory therapist and three ER physicians (including me) converged on him. One nurse got up on a stepstool and started doing CPR. Another put ECG leads on the man's chest and fired up the cardiac monitor and defibrillator. One physician and the RT intubated the patient. The other physician brought a portable ultrasound machine to scan the heart.

"What's the patient's name?" I asked Charlie, a paramedic I recognized.

"His name is Moon," he said. "His family is from South Korea."

"Did someone call them? They need to know what's happening."

"The person at the gym got hold of the family," Charlie explained. "He lives with his mother and a younger brother. They're on the way."

At that point, Moon's chances of surviving were dismal. In 2024, *BMJ* published the results of a large American study that looked at nearly 350,000 adult patients who had a cardiac arrest and received CPR in hospital from 2000 to 2021. The study was led by Masashi Okubo, assistant professor in the Department of Emergency Medicine at the University of Pittsburgh School of Medicine. A colleague of mine, Dr. Laurie Morrison, an ER physician at Toronto's Sunnybrook Health Sciences Centre, was a co-author.

The researchers looked at the duration of CPR and its impact on immediate survival and favourable neurological outcome. What they found tracks with our frontline experience. Beyond thirty-two minutes of CPR, fewer than one per cent of patients emerge as they were prior to their heart stoppage.

The goal of the study, the authors wrote, was to "provide resuscitation teams, patients, and their surrogates with insights into the likelihood of favorable outcomes if the patient continues to receive cardiopulmonary resuscitation beyond that time point." Frontline healthcare providers like me have become increasingly aware of the costs of continuing CPR and advanced cardiac life support (ACLS) when those efforts are likely to be futile.

Moon had by that point been in cardiac arrest well beyond that threshold.

"Listen up," I said. "Moon has been down for over forty minutes. I suggest we continue CPR and ACLS long enough to do a bedside ultrasound to assess the heart, but if there's no cardiac activity, I'm calling it. Any objections?"

A couple of people exhaled loudly, but there were no objections. You may be wondering why I didn't wait to ask the family for permission to stop resuscitation. The decision to stop a Code Blue is made by the healthcare team. It's based on factors like how long the patient has not had a return of normal heart rhythm and blood pressure. There are legal cases in which the decision to stop resuscitation has been challenged by survivors, but in general, families do not have the authority to override the medical team's decision.

One of the ER physicians wheeled the ultrasound machine right next to Moon, put gel on the probe and placed the probe on the left side of the chest.

"Stop CPR," I said to the nurse.

The display showed a good view of the heart. It wasn't moving.

Just then, a nurse appeared at the door to the resuscitation room. "Excuse me, everyone," she said. "I have Moon's mother and brother, and I'd like to bring them in."

"This is exactly the right moment for that," I said.

"This is Sook Park, Moon's mother," said the nurse as she led the woman in. "And this is Moon's brother, Saja."

Everyone in the room stopped what they were doing.

"Sook, Saja, I'm Dr. Goldman. I'm the doctor in charge. I want to explain what's been going on," I said to them. "Moon's heart stopped at the gym. The manager called 911 and started CPR. The paramedics took over and worked very hard on Moon for the past forty or forty-five minutes. They gave him medications that shocked his heart several times to try to restart it. They got the heart back to normal rhythm, but it's no longer beating."

"Please save my son," said Sook.

"We have tried our best, but we can't save Moon at this point," I told her gently. "I'm sorry that we weren't able to do that."

"Can't we do anything?" Saja asked.

"When someone dies, the hearing is the last thing to go," I told them. "You can tell Moon how much you love him."

Sook wept softly as she grabbed tightly onto the son she had held since birth. "Please don't die."

"We love you, Moon," said Saja. Then he turned to me. "Did my brother suffer?"

"I don't think so."

"Can we get a couple of chairs for Sook and Saja to sit on?" I said. "We're going to stop what we're doing now and clear the room. I want to thank everyone who came to help out." Then, turning my attention back to Moon's devastated mother and brother, I said, "I'm sure there are lots of things you want to say to him. Take as much time as you need."

A while later, I returned to the resuscitation room to talk more with Moon's family. As I entered, I saw Sook holding Moon's lifeless hand. Saja had his hand on his mother's upper back.

"I'm sorry to interrupt," I said, "but there's something important I need to ask the two of you. Has anyone else in the family died young like Moon?"

"My baby brother died when he was sixteen," said Sook.

Saja looked stunned. "I had an uncle?"

"It happened so long ago," said Sook. "For a long time, I thought our family was cursed. Now I'm sure of it."

"Not cursed," I told her. "But there may be a connection between Moon's death and your brother's."

There are several possible causes of sudden cardiac death in young adults. The most common is hypertrophic cardiomyopathy. This is a condition in which the heart muscle becomes thickened without an obvious cause such as severe high blood pressure or a stenotic, or tight, heart valve. Another is long QT syndrome, which affects the repolarization, or resetting, of the heart after an electrical heartbeat. The underlying condition, which can be congenital, causes the QT interval (as seen on an ECG) to be excessively long. It's linked to unexplained fainting and sudden death, especially in young people. These episodes can be triggered by exercise or stress.

But what was on my mind was Brugada syndrome, a very rare

condition that affects three to five people per 10,000. The disorder predisposes people to heart rhythm disturbances that can trigger sudden death. It's been called sudden unexplained nocturnal death syndrome because people with it often die in their sleep. Brugada syndrome is eight to ten times more common in men than women, and it's also more prevalent in males of Southeast Asian descent. It's an autosomal dominant condition, meaning first-degree relatives of patients who have the disease are also at risk.

Brugada syndrome can be diagnosed by an ECG. The cure is an implantable cardioverter-defibrillator, or ICD. Current recommendations are to insert an ICD in patients who survive cardiac arrest and patients with ECG abnormalities who faint, or have an episode of "syncope," as such episodes are referred to clinically. The condition can also be treated by radio frequency ablation, which is a procedure in which high-frequency radio waves that generate heat are used to ablate, or destroy, tissue in the front part of the right ventricle. Ablation has been found to prevent sudden death due to ventricular fibrillation in patients with symptomatic Brugada syndrome.

"Saja, the fact that your brother and your uncle both died suddenly makes me concerned that you have the same condition. I'm going to suggest that we do an ECG right now."

It turned out Saja had the same ECG abnormality as Moon. I referred him to a cardiologist who specializes in heart rhythm disturbances. Eventually, he got an ICD and is doing well.

Like I said, bad things can happen to young patients. But sometimes, good can come from the bad.

I dare say every frontline healthcare provider I know has a story or two about a young patient and some sort of catastrophe. Many of those stories—not surprisingly—involve accidents. Statistics Canada says that among young adults, unintentional injuries are the leading cause of death and one of the leading causes of hospitalizations.

Dawn Gavin knows all about that. The sixty-eight-year-old has been a registered nurse since 1978 and a triage nurse at Halifax's Queen Elizabeth II Health Sciences Centre on and off since 2015. Like a lot of other people who work in the ER, Dawn calls herself an adrenaline junkie.

One shift, she recalls working triage when a young man was brought to the ER by his girlfriend. He had been driving an all-terrain vehicle and had got caught with a rope and flipped over the windshield and the handlebars. "He didn't look well," Dawn told me. "I did an assessment, and his blood pressure was low, [but] his heart rate was okay."

Dawn thought the young man was in shock from internal injuries. She talked to the team leader, who agreed to put the patient in a trauma bay. Once he was flat on a stretcher, his blood pressure rose and he looked more comfortable. So comfortable, in fact, that the ER physician wondered if his initial low blood pressure was due not to shock but to something called vasovagal syncope. This is a minor condition in which certain triggers, such as the sight of blood or extreme emotional distress, cause your heart rate and blood pressure to drop suddenly. That leads to reduced blood flow to your brain, causing you to briefly lose consciousness.

The ER doctor told Dawn he was planning to observe the young man for an hour and send him home if he remained stable. Dawn was alarmed by this plan. "He's compromised," she told the doctor, "and when he crashes, he'll burn." She urged him to get a CT scan to look for internal injuries. "If you haven't done a CT scan, you'll have to deal with me in person," she warned without a trace of nurse-speak. Dawn's seniority and her years of experience meant she could speak more bluntly to the doctors, and they would listen.

And what happened to the young man? Dawn said the doctor

took her advice and got the scan, which showed massive and irreparable damage to the spleen and the small intestine. Fifteen minutes later, "the guy was in the OR and he had lost twenty-five inches of bowel and his spleen." But he survived.

Dawn doesn't see that episode as vindication for her instincts. "It's very humbling at times, because you still make mistakes, and you learn," she told me. "You learn something new every day. But I think the big thing is advocating for patients."

Not every bad thing that happens to young patients is caused by trauma. Some are caused by illnesses that tend to affect older patients, like coronary artery disease, and some are due to serious infections.

Sometimes young people with life-threatening ailments present in very bizarre ways. Dr. Amy Nason of the QEII in Halifax told me about one night shift when a man in his early twenties came to the ER coughing up blood. The technical term for that is hemoptysis. It tends to happen when the lung tissue or the bronchial passages are damaged or inflamed. Some of the most common causes of hemoptysis are bronchitis, pneumonia, tuberculosis, chronic obstructive pulmonary disease and heart failure. In an older patient who has a long history of cigarette smoking, lung cancer would be high on the list of ominous possibilities.

Nason told me how she thought through the case. "He's young, in his early twenties," she recalled. "He looked well . . . and gave a story that was more like pneumonia. Had a cough and fever. Pretty common." She ordered a chest X-ray to look for a patch of pneumonia.

Suddenly, she was summoned back to the patient's bedside because he'd started coughing up copious quantities of blood. "It is a large volume, like three hundred to five hundred millilitres," she remembered. "He was just coughing up clot after clot after clot." Realizing that something wasn't adding up, she turned to look at the patient's chest X-ray—and her eyes went wide. "He's got a huge lesion in his chest and it looks almost like a doughnut."

We call these "cavitary lung lesions." That's an X-ray term for an abnormality defined by a lucent, or dark, area in the centre completely surrounded by a large white area. One of the most common causes of a cavitary lung lesion like that is tuberculosis, and this patient did have risk factors for that. "He'd lived on a reserve in Manitoba . . . and didn't seek a lot of medical care," Nason said. "He comes from a place where TB is endemic."

TB would have been the easy conclusion to draw, but it turns out that certain cancers found in the chest cavity can look very similar. Nason decided to confer with the radiology resident on call.

"He's like, 'What's going on with his testicles?'" Nason told me. She was dumbfounded. To make certain she understood him, the resident repeated himself. "You should ask him about his testicles, for sure."

She marched to the patient's room and asked if anything was going on with his testicles. Bingo! The patient admitted that he had felt a lump in his scrotum for some time but, as a university student, hadn't got around to getting it checked out.

Nason asked if she could examine him. "Sure enough, he had a big testicular tumour," she said. That meant the lesion in his lung wasn't TB but a cancer metastasis. Not the usual way of making that diagnosis. "Typically, we pick up testicular cancer with testicular exams or ultrasounds," she said. "It was a wild and fabulous pickup for a radiology resident who that night was thinking, 'Why does a young guy have a big lesion in his chest?'"

The overall prognosis for testicular cancer is excellent. Treatment is successful in more than 95 per cent of cases. Even cancer that has spread to the lungs has at least intermediate prospects for survival. And that was the case for this young man.

"He did great," said Nason. "He had his testicle removed. He went on to do chemo and radiation for his lung disease. I've seen him since for a completely unrelated complaint."

Although testicular cancer is not all that common—just one in every 250 men will be diagnosed with the disease during their lifetime—it is one of the most common cancers in younger men. But lately, younger patients have also been getting a far greater share of cancers that we usually see in their parents and grandparents.

2:15 a.m.

My heart sinks as soon as I open the first few images of Rodrigo's CT scan. Where the sigmoid colon meets the rectum, there's a tumour the size of a large grapefruit. It nearly fills the inside of the bowel and has penetrated the wall. A smorgasbord of white-and-grey dappled bits of tumour cram the inside of the belly cavity between loops of small intestine, and there are also four chunks of tumour inside the liver. It's like no body part has been spared. Even the bottoms of Rodrigo's lungs, such as I'm able to see on this abdominal CT scan, are full of cancer.

How the heck am I supposed to have a conversation like that in a chaotic place like this?

We do have a method, thanks to my late friend and colleague the British physician Dr. Robert Buckman. Buckman was a well-known cancer specialist and the author of fourteen books and dozens of articles that dealt with cancer, general health and death. He was also an expert in the doctor-patient relationship, particularly when it came to breaking bad news.

In the late 1990s, Buckman collaborated with Dr. Walter Baile, a psychiatrist and professor at the University of Texas MD Anderson Cancer Center in Houston, to develop the SPIKES protocol, a six-step framework to help frontline health professionals communicate complex and difficult information to patients and their families.

SPIKES is an acronym for setting, perspective, invitation, knowledge, empathy, and strategy and summary. "Setting" is a reminder to find an appropriate space to hold a sensitive discussion. Buckman and Baile argue that this is critical no matter how full and frantic the ER happens to be. "While private spaces can be scarce in a busy ED," they write, "every attempt should be made to find a quiet area, especially if the patient is in a curtained room or shared space. If they are in a hallway bed, discussions can be held in private care rooms, triage rooms, or quiet alcoves."

"Perspective" means trying to grasp what patients and their family members understand about the situation being discussed. "Invitation" means asking for permission to share the news with family members and to what extent. "Knowledge" means tailoring the information to each patient's level of understanding. "Empathy" means tracking verbal and non-verbal cues to be aware of what patients and their families are going through as they process the information. And finally, "strategy and summary" means recapping the information shared while discussing a clear plan for what comes next.

Before heading to Rodrigo's cubicle, I make a pit stop at triage and hand my phone over to Samir. I don't want to be distracted or look like I'm too busy to talk.

It's going to be one of those conversations.

"Rodrigo, sorry it's taken a while to get the report of the CT scan." A million thoughts run through my mind. He and Christine are about to get the most shocking and terrible news imaginable. I close the door as slowly as I can and grab a seat on the stretcher. I'm aware that they're looking at me.

When I was much younger, I dreaded giving bad news because I feared sounding glib or being blamed. Now I understand that my job isn't to get myself through this terrible moment. It's to get them through it.

"There's a lot of technical language I have to translate from the report," I begin. "Before I get into that, I want to find out how much detail you want me to go into."

"All of it," says Christine.

"Rodrigo, how about you?"

"Something's wrong with me and I want to get better," he says, looking at his wife.

"The news isn't good," I begin.

Rodrigo looks concerned. Christine looks like she's been expecting me to say this.

"We found a tumour in your rectum," I continue. "It's in the lowest part of your abdomen."

"You're saying it's cancer?" Rodrigo asks.

"Yes, it's cancer," I tell them.

Christine starts to cry. Rodrigo reaches out for her hand.

"There's more to tell you," I say. "The cancer has spread to your liver and into your abdomen. That's why you're having so much pain."

"You're saying it's . . . it's . . ." Christine struggles to find the word that's entered the vernacular.

"Metastasized," I offer. "Yes. That's what's happening inside you, Rodrigo. I'm so sorry to be telling you this awful news."

"But I have constipation," says Rodrigo. "I have hemorrhoids. That's what my doctor told me."

"I told you to ask if it could be cancer." Christine sounds angry.

"I did!" Rodrigo is trying desperately to process what I'm telling him. "My doctor said I was too young to have colon cancer."

"That's what a lot of people think," I try to explain. "Even doctors."

"What happens next?" Rodrigo asks.

"In my judgment, you're too ill to go home," I reply. "With your permission, I'd like to refer you to the internal medicine team on call so they can admit you to the hospital. I can keep you comfortable while you wait to be seen. Once you're admitted, they'll need to do more CT scans, an MRI and blood tests to figure out what stage of cancer you've got and how to treat it."

"Is he going to live?" Christine asks.

"I'm not a cancer specialist and I don't have detailed information about that," I reply carefully. "The cancer specialist will recommend treatments that should help shrink the cancer—maybe even to the point at which surgery is possible. But when colon cancer spreads to the liver and the abdomen, it becomes very difficult to cure."

"Our son is four years old," says Rodrigo.

That lands between us very hard.

Christine and Rodrigo are looking at each other.

"You're going to beat this," she tells her husband.

Colorectal cancer is common and deadly. The Canadian Cancer Society says it's the second leading cause of cancer deaths in men and the third leading cause in women. Long thought of as a disease of older Canadians, it's been showing up with more frequency in younger people like Rodrigo.

It's a trend that emergency physicians like Dr. Keerat Grewal are noticing. As noted earlier, Grewal has a Canadian Institutes of Health Research project grant to lead a multidisciplinary study looking at patients in Ontario who are diagnosed with cancer in the ER. In addition, Grewal and her team combed the ICES clinical database for every patient in Ontario with a confirmed diagnosis of cancer to see how many of them were seen in an ER in the ninety days before they had a biopsy.

Grewal says ER physicians are seeing many patients of all ages with cancer. Some are young. In the ICES study, she says, "we didn't look at the age of the patients, but I'd say anecdotally, you're seeing younger and younger patients with cancer who are already on treatment. With GI cancers, you don't start screening until you're fifty. But I've either diagnosed or seen patients admitted with confirmed cancer who are younger than the fifty-year-old cutoff."

Cancer specialists like Dr. Sharlene Gill, a professor of medicine at the University of British Columbia and an oncologist at BC Cancer, have also reported seeing younger patients with colorectal cancer. "I've been treating colorectal cancer for over twenty years, and no doubt we are seeing patients being diagnosed at an earlier age," she told my colleague Brandie Weikle on *White Coat, Black Art*.

Behind the anecdotes is some alarming data. A study published in 2020 in the journal *Cancer* by epidemiologist Emily Heer and colleagues found that between 1983 and 2012, among people under the age of fifty, rates increased significantly for thirteen kinds of cancer, including colon, breast, kidney, pancreas and thyroid. Their analysis found that the most dramatic increase was for colorectal cancers in people ages twenty to thirty-nine. In that age group, there was a fivefold increase in rectal cancer and a twofold increase in colon cancer. Among twenty- to twenty-four-year-olds, rates of colorectal cancers increased 4 to 6 per cent a year. Among thirty- to thirty-nine-year-olds, there were also significant increases for pancreatic cancer.

A 2022 paper published in the journal *Current Oncology* discovered a paradox: Rates of colon cancer in people over fifty in Canada and other developed countries are declining. Compared with older Canadians, those born after 1980 are two to two and a half times more likely to be diagnosed with colon cancer in middle age and younger. Experts aren't sure why this is, but given the speed with which this trend has taken hold, it's unlikely that genetic factors are at work. Researchers are looking at factors such as diet, obesity, lack of exercise, tobacco and alcohol use and environmental risks such as exposure to chemicals.

The US has also seen some startling increases in rates of cancer in younger people. In 2023, the American Cancer Society reported that in 2019, 20 per cent of all colon and rectal cancers were found in patients under fifty-five years of age. That figure is double the rate of those cancers in younger people seen in 1983. That prompted both the United States Preventive Services Task Force and the Multi-Society Task Force on Colorectal Cancer to recommend that most Americans be screened for colorectal cancer starting at age forty-five, five years earlier than previously recommended.

As of now, the minimum age for screening in Canada is fifty, but Bishop Brigante campaigned hard to lower it to forty-five. That's how old he was when he was diagnosed with stage 4 colorectal cancer.

Brigante was a Scarborough-born hip-hop artist and actor who became known within the hip-hop community as a maven of battle rap. Bishop was diagnosed with colorectal cancer in October 2023, but his symptoms began two years earlier. He complained to various doctors that he was having abdominal pain, diarrhea and blood in his stool.

"My doctors would say, 'That's hemorrhoids.' They told me that I had irritable bowel syndrome . . . I was told, 'You just gotta kind of work on your diet, fix the food you eat and stuff like that,'" Bishop told me.

By the time he got a colonoscopy plus CTs and MRIs, his cancer had metastasized. The five-year survival for stage 4 colon cancer is between 11.1 and 13.4 per cent.

What did stage 4 mean to Brigante?

"I know it's dangerous, I know it's scary," he said. "But could it have been avoided? Yeah."

It's the avoidance part that turned Bishop into an advocate for early detection of colorectal cancer regardless of age. As part of his public advocacy, Bishop started a petition at Change.org seeking to lower the age criterion for colonoscopies from fifty to thirty. As of this writing, the petition had more than 38,000 signatures.

"It's very simple," he told me. "I want to save lives. I found a purpose because I felt that there is a broken system. An outdated system and an outdated way of looking at certain things."

Bishop died on March 30, 2025, at the age of forty-six. His petition lives on in his memory, and his allies in the public and inside the medical community are carrying on the fight to lower the age for colorectal cancer screening.

Dr. Sharlene Gill told me, "I do feel that we need to, in Canada, look very seriously at lowering our age of screening to forty-five."

As ERs see more and more younger people getting diagnosed with colorectal cancer, it's clear to me that the system needs to adapt. One hospital making an effort to do that is Sunnybrook Health Sciences Centre, in Toronto. In early 2019, the hospital opened its Young Adult Colorectal Cancer Clinic, the first clinic in Canada that focuses on treating colorectal cancer patients under fifty years of age. The clinic is run by family doctor Petra Wildgoose and surgical oncologist Shady Ashamalla.

"The aim of the clinic is to address the complex and unique needs of young adults under age 50 who have been diagnosed with colorectal cancer, and the concerns they have to live with in the decades after having had that diagnosis," Dr. Wildgoose said in an article posted to the hospital's website. The clinic has assembled a multidisciplinary team of oncologists, social workers, psychologists and geneticists and a nurse navigator. These people work together to help younger patients deal with issues that older patients may not have, such as fertility problems, young children at home, challenges at work and concerns about hereditary cancer.

I make a mental note to tell the general internal medicine team admitting Rodrigo about the clinic at Sunnybrook. I hope he lives long enough to benefit from it.

2:35 a.m.

Paramedics lift Britany's stretcher onto the back of an ambulance. She has IVs in both arms and looks like she's been swallowed up by a big orange blanket. A middle-aged woman dressed in street clothes hops into the ambulance after her and holds her hand. I assume it's her mother.

A cardiovascular surgeon at a hospital across the city has accepted Britany. Ahu is accompanying her. It's Ahu's first medical transport. She's excited about getting some real-world experience, but more importantly, she's worried about her patient.

"Got everything you need?" I ask her. I already know the answer.

Ahu shows me four colour-coded syringes. "Labetalol to lower the blood pressure, phenylephrine in case her blood pressure crashes," she says, leading me a few steps away from the ambulance and out of Britany's earshot. "Ketamine to sedate her and rocuronium to paralyze her in case I need to intubate."

"And," I add, "you've got two hands in case you need to do CPR plus an oropharyngeal airway and bag valve mask in case you need to ventilate in a hurry. Never forget the basics."

"I won't," says Ahu as a paramedic helps her into the back of the ambulance.

Just as the ambulance doors are about to close, she turns back to me. "While I'm gone, can you check on a patient I just saw? She's a thirty-one-year-old woman with a history of kidney stones. She says she had another one five days ago. She went to another ER with typical pain. I ordered a CT scan."

"Will do," I tell her.

"I'm kind of worried about her," says Ahu. "She looks sick. A wise doctor once told me that bad things happen to young patients too."

A paramedic closes the door to the ambulance. They pop the lights and sirens as they drive off.

It's both rewarding and sobering to have the lessons you teach residents given back to you.

CHAPTER NINE

AN ER ON WHEELS

2:45 a.m.

"Brian, I'm glad I saw you," says Virginia, the paramedic who brought Molly to the ER a few hours ago. She and her partner, Tom, wheel in a young woman who is shaking and whose complexion appears flushed. "How's Molly doing?"

"She had surgery to remove her ruptured ectopic pregnancy and fallopian tube," I reply. "She's in the ICU and is expected to make a full recovery."

"Thanks to you and your portable ultrasound machine," Virginia tells me. "It would come in handy for those times when I have trouble finding a vein to put in an IV. Some of the paramedics have taken an ultrasound course."

"I think that's a fantastic idea," I tell her. Turning to the patient, I ask, "Who have you brought to the ER this time?"

"Circe is a thirty-two-year-old with fever of forty degrees Celsius and rigors," Virginia tells me. Rigors are a sudden feeling of cold with shivering, closely followed by a rise in temperature. It's often an indicator of a potentially serious bacterial infection in the bloodstream. "She's also complaining of severe pain in her chest."

"What have you done for her?" I ask.

"We started an IV and a bolus of fluids. Since Circe qualified for the PITSTOP clinical trial, we gave her an intramuscular injection of either the antibiotic ceftriaxone or a placebo."

PITSTOP stands for Paramedic Initiated Treatment of Sepsis Targeting Out-of-hospital Patients, a research project designed to see whether paramedics can save more lives by giving certain patients intravenous fluids and an intramuscular injection of ceftriaxone, a powerful antibiotic used to treat sepsis caused by serious conditions such as pneumonia and kidney infections.

"You don't know whether Circe got the real deal or the placebo," I reply.

"That's right. But if she's unstable, we can break the code and find out which she got," says Virginia. "So far, her vitals have been rock-solid."

"Let's hope things stay that way." I tell Virginia and Tom to wheel Circe to the triage area.

I love the idea of expanding the paramedic toolkit. Gone are the days when the most salient thing they did was bring patients to the ER. I've seen paramedics deliver primary care and even palliative care in patients' homes. And there's much more they can do to save lives by starting treatment in the field, rather than waiting until they arrive in the ER. Sometimes that delay can be the difference between life and death. I also believe we can achieve better results if we get more doctors like me out of the ER to deal with emergencies where they happen.

There's an ER physician in BC who is showing us how to do just that.

Air Canada Express was an hour late getting me into the West Kootenay Regional Airport in Castlegar, BC, but as I gazed out over the tall, majestic mountains and picturesque yet narrow valleys, I felt my stress fade away. It could have been worse. The surrounding terrain and microclimate make the airport challenging to land at on the best days, and any hint of bad weather means pilots won't even be cleared to try. That's why the airport has the unflattering nickname of Cancelgar.

But on this day, we touched down with no problems, and I strolled past the small terminal building's baggage carousel and was almost halfway to the sliding exit doors when I spotted a man in his forties strutting towards me. He was about five foot ten with a perfectly shaved head and a wide, toothy grin. As he approached me, other passengers and airport employees turned to gawk at him—and not just because he was wearing a conspicuous orange jumpsuit festooned with lots of reflective patches and even more gadgets. Dr. Nic Sparrow, the most overqualified first responder in Canada, has fans.

"Promote the heck out of this guy," said Kevin Benson, a retired firefighter from Yellowknife who recognized Nic when he came to the airport to pick up an arriving passenger. "We need him national. In rural areas, he's essential. As a firefighter, we sometimes can't get to places quick enough. And he can."

Sparrow is an emergency medical services (EMS) physician who until quite recently worked in the ER at the Castlegar and District Community Health Centre and at the Kootenay Lake Hospital in nearby Nelson. Now he works full-time as a community response doctor for the Kootenay Emergency Response Physicians Association, or KERPA, a charitable organization he founded in 2014. KERPA's mandate is to help critically ill and injured patients throughout the Kootenay region by responding to 911 calls where there's an immediate threat to life. Sparrow is one of a very small number of MDs in Canada who respond to EMS calls in the field.

Sparrow traces his passion for emergency medicine to a near tragedy at a very young age: When he was just five years old, his two-year-old sister, Madeline, almost died. In England, where

Sparrow was born and raised, he and his family were at a Red Cross garden party when Maddie got out of her stroller and wandered off unnoticed. A friend of little Nic's mother's found the toddler face-down in a pond, blue in the face and in cardiac arrest. "I still remember the screams from my mom," Sparrow told me. Very quickly, a Red Cross first-aider pulled her out and started CPR. Paramedics and police were called, and Maddie was soon transported to the nearest hospital. She survived without brain damage, and today she's married with two kids of her own. The local newspaper dubbed her "Miraculous Maddie."

Not surprisingly, the incident stuck in the young boy's mind, and when he grew up, he decided to become a doctor. "At a very young age, I saw how skilled action at the scene of an incident can have a massive impact on the outcomes of the patient, and the outcomes of everyone who loves and cares for that person," Sparrow says on the KERPA website. "Starting KERPA came from a place of knowing that having a trained pre-hospital provider, in the right place at the right time, could help critically ill or injured patients have the very best chance of survival."

Sparrow earned his MBBS—bachelor of medicine, bachelor of surgery, and the British equivalent of an MD—at Imperial College in London, then trained at St. Mary's Hospital in Paddington. The hospital is the major trauma centre for northwest London and runs a twenty-four-hour accident and emergency department. Later, Nic spent time working as a trauma physician in Johannesburg, South Africa. Those experiences made him accustomed to being part of a dedicated EMS unit. "The UK and the European model is that physicians across the country would be available to respond to critical calls [in the field] in any region," he explained to me. "In the UK, it's a given that there are physicians across the country on call to come and help." In his drive to become one of those physicians, Sparrow got extra field training in the UK.

In 2008, he moved to Canada and began to practise family medicine at a clinic in Gibsons, a coastal community of just under 5,000 people along the Georgia Strait in southwestern BC. To his surprise, he soon discovered that physicians in Canada do not act as first responders, resuscitating sick and injured patients at emergency scenes. "I was kind of like, 'Wow! Why is this not part of the EMS system in North America?'" Sparrow said.

One day in March 2009, he was at the clinic when he heard several emergency vehicles pass by outside. "I felt like I needed to help." Armed with his emergency field training and his trauma experience in the UK and South Africa, he got in his car and followed the sirens to Good Samaritan Christenson Village, where he learned that a care home resident had shot at staff members. Sparrow treated one of the shooting victims and later asked BC Emergency Health Services if they would designate him a community response physician. They agreed and even gave him a pager.

"I started volunteering my time," Sparrow said, responding to emergency calls in his own truck, equipped with supplies he'd paid for out of his own pocket. Today, he considers what he did on the Sunshine Coast a pilot program for KERPA.

In 2013, Sparrow and his family moved to Nelson. "I had a friend who said, 'Hey, you should come to Nelson and check it out,'" he told me. He did a locum, or a temporary stint, as an ER physician at the Kootenay Lake Hospital and, he said, "just loved it." Before he knew it, he was looking for a full-time emergency job in the town.

As soon as he and his family were established in Nelson, he began responding to field calls in his own vehicle, just as he had in Gibsons.

Sparrow and I climbed into the Ford Tahoe that serves as his mobile headquarters. It was painted bright orange like his jumpsuit and had a white-on-black KERPA sign and logo on the side. Toronto Paramedic Services provided the Tahoe to KERPA.

"This fully decked out EMS vehicle is carrying probably about $150,000 to $200,000 worth of medical gear inside," Sparrow said proudly. That buys a lot of medical gear: video laryngoscope, automated chest compression device, portable ventilator, portable ultrasound, pelvic binders for trauma patients in shock, chest tubes and vacuum drainage for patients with punctured lungs. And that's all in addition to the standard devices found on paramedic vehicles, like a cardiac monitor, external defibrillator, and bag valve mask. There were also lots of medications, including ones not administered by paramedics, like the paralyzing drug rocuronium for intubations. Think of the vehicle as a resuscitation room on wheels.

Along with the extra equipment comes specialized training. Unlike me, Sparrow has completed a course in pre-hospital trauma life support, which teaches providers how to rapidly assess a trauma patient in the field and minimize delays in initiating transport. He's also taken the Neonatal Resuscitation Program and courses in pediatric and adult advanced life support (ALS). He's even completed the Tactical Emergency Casualty Care program, which teaches frontline providers how to apply lessons from the military to the civilian world of tactical medicine.

"And then obviously," Sparrow said, "[I have] on-the-road experience responding to critical calls to be oriented to all the equipment that we carry and know how to use it in remote, rural austere environments."

There are lots of remote and rural austere environments in the Kootenay region, which covers 7.6 million hectares of the southeast corner of British Columbia. It extends from the Alberta border in the east to the Arrow Lakes country in the west and from Kinbasket Lake in the north to the US border in the south.

Sparrow explained that most of his emergency calls are in Nelson and Castlegar, but he has also responded to calls in smaller and more remote communities like Salmo and Winlaw, as well as in Kaslo, a village on the west shore of Kootenay Lake, at least a two-hour drive from Castlegar. "And on a few occasions," he told me, "we've been placed in helicopters and flown even further to help."

I asked him how many kilometres he puts on the Tahoe each year. "Probably 15,000 to 20,000," he said as he stared out the windshield. "This is Highway 3 that we're driving on. It goes all the way from Hope, BC, to Medicine Hat, Alberta, which is about 840 kilometres." For comparison's sake, the entire length of Great Britain, from the northern tip of Scotland to the southern coast of England, is 1,000 kilometres. "So this is a huge stretch of highway going across a huge amount of BC."

Huge and sparsely populated. "The advanced life support paramedics and critical care paramedics are situated in busy centres and cities," Sparrow said. "We do have an ALS unit running out of Trail. But all the time that KERPA has been operating, there has been no advanced life support readily available in the Nelson area."

Suddenly, our travelogue was interrupted by a page from the ambulance service. "This is a chest pain call," Sparrow explained, "so we'll call dispatch and just find out whether we're required."

He found a safe place to pull over so he could call the local dispatcher on his cellphone.

"Hey, it's Dr. Nic from KERPA in Nelson," he said. "Happy to respond. Just need the address." He pulled a pen and a small notebook from the top pocket on his orange coveralls and made some notes. "Can you spell the last name for me?"

When Sparrow finished his call, he filled me in. The patient, he said, was a male having palpitations, chest pain and maybe alcohol withdrawal. We were a little over 17 kilometres from the man's home. Sparrow flicked on the Tahoe's emergency lights and sirens and accelerated to 120 in a 90-kilometre zone. I've never done something like that before and was fascinated by how much thought he put into speeding safely. Unsurprisingly, he has taken a course in operating emergency vehicles.

"How do you feel as you're heading to an emergency?" I asked him. "Are you an adrenaline junkie?"

"I don't always enjoy going to calls," he replied, "but I feel like my calling in life is sometimes to be in some really chaotic situations and maybe bring some sort of peace to the storm, if you know what I mean. And just be there to help people."

We pulled up at the scene and parked close to an ambulance. Sparrow opened the back of his Tahoe and grabbed his trauma backpack, crammed with resuscitation gear. A paramedic filled him in. The patient, he said, was "ticking along."

"It's probably more dehydration, throwing up," Nic concluded. "We've got the monitors. We'll have a quick look."

I followed Sparrow into the young man's modest and sparsely furnished apartment living room. The man was sitting on a mattress on the floor. He looked like he was in his late twenties or early thirties and seemed in distress.

Sparrow introduced himself to the man. "I'm one of the doctors responding alongside the ambulance service. I'm just going to place you on a monitor and we're going to check your heart out. Can you tell me what's been happening today?"

"Fair amount of drinking," mumbled the young man.

While Sparrow did his assessment, I talked to Len Coates, a volunteer firefighter based in Castlegar. Coates told me that sometimes firefighters, paramedics and Sparrow all receive a call for medical assistance. Who gets there first depends on which units are available and where they happen to be, but Sparrow, he said, brings things to each call that other first responders cannot because he has a scope of practice beyond that of paramedics.

"He is able to put an intravenous in with certain medications that paramedics cannot," said Coates. "He has an ultrasound as well, so he can literally see what is taking place with the patient. [Because he's] able to do stuff on scene, he's able to delay, or slow down the clock, so that there's time to get the patient to the hospital. And that's a big thing in rural communities, especially."

Coates told me that he's seen Sparrow make a big difference in several emergency situations. "There's been a number of motor vehicle accidents that he's been to where he has helped save people's lives," he said. "People catching their arms or legs in things and possibly bleeding out. He's able to help stop the bleeding and ensure that the person is able to make it to the hospital while we work on a vehicle to get that person out. That's one of the biggest things that we see."

I glanced over at Sparrow, who signalled that he'd finished his assessment of the patient. We made our way back to the Tahoe, where he wiped down his equipment with disinfectant. Then we followed the ambulance bearing the patient to the ER at the Castlegar Health Centre. On the way, Sparrow offered a debrief.

"The patient had fast heart rate, nausea and vomiting associated with alcohol withdrawal," he said. "We did a twelve-lead ECG, simply because he was having some chest discomfort, probably from the vomiting. That was nice and normal. Checked his blood sugar. We'll follow the paramedics in just because he has a history of alcohol withdrawal seizures [and] we're carrying the medication to be able to stop that. The paramedics will put an IV in and give some anti-sickness medication, and then we'll go from there."

An alcohol withdrawal seizure is not a trivial medical problem. It's a possible symptom of delirium tremens—also called DTs or alcohol withdrawal delirium. It's an uncommon but severe type of alcohol withdrawal that typically begins forty-eight to seventy-two hours after a sudden stop to drinking or a dramatic reduction in alcohol intake caused by abdominal pain or vomiting

Alcohol is a depressant to the brain, but the brain builds up a tolerance to the depressant effects by raising levels of a stimulating chemical called glutamate. When you stop drinking suddenly, you get a spike in glutamate, which overstimulates the brain, causing symptoms such as an extreme rise in blood pressure, tremors, severe excitability and seizures. The mortality rate for delirium tremens with prompt recognition and treatment is between 5 and 15 per cent. Without medical attention, the mortality rate is around 37 per cent. Treatment involves intravenous fluids, thiamine and benzodiazepines to relieve symptoms and stop seizures.

If this patient had been having seizures and other symptoms of severe alcohol withdrawal, Sparrow could have administered the short-acting intravenous benzodiazepine midazolam in the field. In the ER we use the same medication to stop epileptic seizures of all kinds. When we see patients who are having seizures, we try to stop them as quickly as possible to avoid a condition called status epilepticus, a medical emergency that starts when a seizure lasts longer than expected (typically longer than five minutes). After that point, it gets harder to stop a seizure with medications. The longer a seizure lasts, the higher the risk of death.

A quick dose of midazolam administered in the field can stop a seizure. Unfortunately, many of the first responders in rural and remote BC are primary care paramedics who are not authorized to administer the medication. "And that's some of the challenge," he explained, "because in a rural area in British Columbia, we don't have many advanced life support resources. In the Nelson area, KERPA was the only resource carrying midazolam and still is currently. So if KERPA is not available, patients could be seizing for over an hour before getting to the hospital." And that, says Sparrow, would more than double the patient's risk of dying.

He pulled up at the Castlegar hospital just as the paramedics were wheeling the patient into the ER.

"What are you bringing for us?" asked a nurse named Joy.

"A thirty-one-year-old male alcohol detox, essentially," Sparrow told her, "and has been detoxing over the last day or two, Lots of nausea, vomiting, just feeling really unwell. Previous history of alcohol seizures."

"When was his last drink?"

"I think it was last night," he replied. "He's had two withdrawal seizures in the past. He hasn't seized [with us] and has been pretty stable. We gave him some [anti-nausea medication] and he's having some fluids. That's really it."

"Okay, perfect. Thanks," said Joy.

That Nic and Joy know one another is hardly surprising. Nurses, doctors and paramedics often develop strong personal relationships. This is especially true in smaller places like Castlegar.

Daniel Leslie also knows Sparrow well. He's a forty-seven-year-old RN who has worked full-time in the Nelson ER for the past seven years. "He's proven himself as an emergency physician," Daniel told me. "He's very calm, he's very clear. He's very good at setting the mood for a critical patient. Very good at establishing an approach for patient care. So we know him as that person that is very professional in his 'emergency physician' life."

Daniel told me that he's known Sparrow for more than a decade—well before he started in the ER. Prior to nursing school, he worked ski patrol and volunteered with search and rescue. "I first interacted with Dr. Sparrow as a team leader responding to an injury at Kootenay Pass," he recalled. A snowboarder had gone into a jump, hit something hard and fallen, sustaining a compound fracture of his lower leg. "I went in with the team and assessed and stabilized the patient," he said. "We ended up having to spend the night on the mountain and I did have some communication [by radio] to Nic, just about the injury and how we should stabilize it."

Daniel noted that the geography of the Kootenay region is the reason a lot of people become patients in the emergency department. "We live in southeast BC. It's rolling old mountains. Lots of mountains for sports . . . Patients we see come in with injuries from biking, hiking and skiing," he said. "We get tree well incidents in which people skiing in deep powder fall into a tree well and are critically injured. We've had, I think, two patients die from that specific issue. You're upside down in a tree well with snow kind of caving in on you. Unless you have someone immediately there to pull you out, you're in a bad way."

Daniel told me that, in his view, Sparrow is made for the Kootenays and for the injured and critically ill patients who require his services, because he is trained in field medicine and knows what to do in rapidly changing circumstances. That he's calm in stressful circumstances is a bonus. "When Nic is involved with KERPA, he will accompany the ambulance from the scene to the hospital," Daniel explained. "Essentially . . . he would be running the incident. He would be making the professional medical decisions for that patient, [and] the ambulance crew would be assisting."

In one recent incident, Daniel said, Sparrow came in with a patient who was found unresponsive at home. It wasn't clear why the patient had collapsed, but he required assistance with his airway and breathing. "Nic accompanied the patient in the ambulance [and helped] with respiration, using a bag valve mask with oxygen flowing through it, essentially breathing for the patient," Daniel explained. Sparrow worked on the man while the paramedics drove to the ER in Nelson, more than an hour's drive away. He was taken straight to the resuscitation room, where Sparrow continued ventilating him, even as he gave a report on what he knew about the patient's condition. "He worked at getting some more IV access so we could give the patient medications," Daniel recalled, "and [he helped] with the logistics of getting the patient onto our hospital bed, removing clothing, making sure that all of the assessments were done in linear fashion . . . [and] that we knew all of the information that he knew would help us care for this patient."

Unfortunately, that patient died. But, Daniel stressed, thanks to Sparrow there have been lots of saves. He said Sparrow never gives up if there's half a chance at survival.

The Nelson–Nelway Highway is one of the prettiest stretches of road in Canada. Between the Salmo River and the Selkirk Mountains, it's hard to know where to pull over and set your gaze first. The highway starts at the Nelway border crossing, near Metaline Falls, Washington, and goes in nearly a straight line northwest towards Nelson.

I was on the highway heading for Apex Precision Fabrication, just outside of Nelson, to meet a man whose foot was saved from amputation because of quick action by Sparrow and KERPA. When I pulled up at the front door, a man in his fifties wearing a light blue T-shirt, tan pants and a green jacket strode out to meet me with a grin on his face and long greying hair poking out from under a pale green baseball cap.

"I'm Mirek Hladik," he said, greeting me with a firm handshake. Then he promptly took off his left shoe and sock and showed me his ankle.

"Damn, that looks good," I had to admit. I could see just the faintest vertical scar running down from the top of Mirek's ankle and the outlines of grafted skin.

"It looks like nothing happened," said Mirek happily. "There was a big opening, and the skin never recovered. I had to get a skin graft done to cover the wound, and that was a long process. But yeah, that worked out pretty good. Functioning ankle and foot. I have ninety per cent range of motion in my ankle, and it hardly hurts."

As Mirek led me indoors to see where he had his accident, I noted that he walks without a limp. "I can mountain bike. I can rock climb," he said. "I had twenty ski days this year. So I'm really fortunate." Once inside, we stopped at a side wall with a large, rectangular trap door at the bottom. Mirek removed the trap door and pointed towards an open dirt basement used to store aluminum sheets and other raw materials.

"That's where it happened," he said.

One day in 2022, Mirek was working in the basement near a stack of concrete panels leaned against a wall. Each panel was five feet by ten feet and weighed eighty pounds.

"They were not balanced," Mirek explained. "So when I actually touched one of the panels, the whole stack released and fell on me." Mirek was trapped under an estimated two tons of stacked concrete. "My head was sticking out," he recalled. "My left leg snapped right off."

He had a compound double fracture at the bottom of his left tibia and fibula at the ankle. "Compound" means the skin was broken, with both bones sticking out. The ankle was also badly dislocated.

Mirek's wife, June, had been outside the building, clearing away debris, but fortunately for her husband, she had come inside to help him right before the accident took place. When she found him, she grabbed a huge pry bar and was able to lift just enough of the weight off Mirek's body that he could crawl out from underneath the concrete.

"All that dirt was going right inside my bones, but I had to get out," Mirek recalled. He used his good foot to extricate himself. "When I actually saw [my ankle], my first thought was that there was a lot of dead stuff. I was convinced I was going to lose it."

June called 911, and in another stroke of luck for Mirek, Sparrow just happened to be on duty.

"It came through as an entrapment call," Sparrow said.

He arrived expecting to have to extricate Mirek from the pile of concrete but was amazed to see that he and June had already accomplished that.

"He's a pretty tough guy," Sparrow told me. "He was fully conscious and had an isolated lower limb injury. That was one of the worst ankle fractures I've ever seen. It was so obvious the bone was sticking out. The foot was kind of pulseless and was going quite pale."

The circulation to Mirek's foot had been cut off. Sparrow started calculating the time in his head. It was a ten- to fifteen-minute ride to the nearest hospital, with no guarantee that the doctor on duty would know what to do to restore the circulation to Mirek's foot. Sparrow quickly realized that saving the foot would come down to him. "I was thinking if we don't get his foot back [in its proper position], it's going to be probably over an hour with no pulses," he said. "I don't think we've even got ten or fifteen minutes to get him to the hospital."

Sparrow may be an ER physician like me, but he's not an orthopedic surgeon. Nevertheless, he decided to operate on Mirek's ankle right then and there.

"With the assistance of the ambulance crew they dragged me . . . to the front of the parking lot," said Mirek, picking up the story. "Nic asked me if I'm okay to do a procedure to speed things up. I said, 'Yeah, you my man. Let's get it done.'"

Sparrow administered ketamine to relieve Mirek's pain and midazolam to sedate him. He irrigated the ankle with litres of sterile salt water to remove debris and dead tissue. Then he set to work putting the ankle into a semblance of a normal anatomical position.

Except he couldn't do it. Not even with the help of the paramedics and firefighters who responded to the call as well.

"His ankle was so severely dislocated that even with a number of us pulling on it, I was unable to get it back," said Sparrow. This was a deal-breaker. If he couldn't put right Mirek's ankle, then he wouldn't be able to get blood flowing back to the foot, and the foot would die.

But Sparrow is a problem solver, which is a hell of a good thing to be when you're in the field and minutes count. He noticed that the skin over Mirek's foot was being tethered by the protruding bone. This was what was blocking the foot from getting back into position. Sparrow decided to cut the skin.

"I actually had to get a scalpel and cut the skin on the side of his leg very gently down to the bone, making sure I wasn't going through anything like vessels or nerves," he told me. "That was the first time I'd ever had to get a scalpel and cut someone's leg to ensure that an ankle would actually go back in, which is kind of strange."

But it worked!

"It went back in and looked normal," he said. "We checked for pulses. He had a good pulse, and the foot started pinking up."

Now that the foot was no longer in danger, Sparrow and the paramedics decided to bypass the hospital in Nelson and take Mirek directly to Trail, where a regional trauma centre is staffed with orthopedic surgeons.

"And they took it from there," said Sparrow.

A few months later, he bumped into Mirek, who explained that he'd had some post-operative complications and had required grafting to cover the skin that Sparrow had cut away to put the foot back in. But otherwise, he said he was doing well.

Mirek wants to raise funds so KERPA can get another vehicle. He has become one of Sparrow's biggest boosters, and it's not hard to understand why.

Virtually no other physician in Canada responds to emergencies in the field like Sparrow does. In the rest of the country, first response is the exclusive purview of paramedics. Which made me wonder just how local paramedics feel about Sparrow joining them on rescues.

Annemarie Perciasepe is a primary care paramedic attached to Station 421 in Nelson. She's been a paramedic in the West Kootenays for ten years and has worked alongside Sparrow and KERPA for eight. She told me that Sparrow was a startling sight the first time she set eyes on him.

"Before he started KERPA in 2014, he would respond in his own personal vehicle," she said. No flashing lights, no sirens. Just Nic in the same silver SUV he used to ferry his family around town. "He has this beautiful bright orange jumpsuit that he wears. It's very similar to the UK model of physicians that join the EMS crews over there. They basically jump out of helicopters wearing the same thing . . . He's very 'high viz.' You can't miss the guy just kind of rocking up and explaining who he is. 'I'm Nic Sparrow and how can I help?'"

Annemarie told me she's responded to roughly one hundred emergencies alongside Sparrow since being posted to Nelson eight years ago. She has lots of stories, but one winter night in particular stands out.

"There was a really bad car accident right around dusk," she told me. "It was getting dark and snowy. It's just you and your partner and the ambulance."

The accident was a head-on crash involving two vehicles, and at least one other vehicle was peripherally involved. A single occupant in one vehicle had been ejected and had life-threatening injuries. Everybody in the other vehicles had minor injuries only.

Annemarie and her partner brought the ejected patient to their ambulance. "This individual had some very serious injuries," she said. "Our biggest concern was that we couldn't secure an airway. There was too much trauma to the face. We were unable to control bleeding in the throat and clear the airways. It was very challenging for us. We couldn't really do what we needed to do."

To make matters worse, by now the roads were blocked with snow and traffic. The ambulance couldn't move, and Annemarie and her partner were concerned that the patient was unstable.

At that moment, Sparrow arrived and joined the battle to save the patient's life.

"We did a full trauma assessment," Annemarie recalled. The patient had obvious facial and head injuries and likely a chest injury as well. What's more, the head injury was making the patient combative and unable to fully cooperate with the rescue.

Right then and there, Sparrow decided to gain control of the situation by performing a rapid sequence intubation, or RSI. This is the same procedure we did with Molly in the ER. It involves sedating, paralyzing and intubating the patient. But in this case, Sparrow planned on doing it in the field.

"He does this all the time in the hospital," Annemarie clarified, "but out in the field, this was the first time he had done something like this with a group of paramedics."

They weren't in the trauma bay of a full-service ER. They were in the back of an ambulance with limited supplies, at night, and off to the side of a blocked highway in the middle of a snowstorm.

Still, Sparrow had the medications he needed to perform the RSI. He just had to be able to deliver them into the patient's body. The quickest way to do that is to find a vein large enough to insert an IV catheter. But with trauma patients in shock, good veins are hard to find. The next best thing is to do what's called an intraosseous, or IO, infusion. You use a small battery-operated power tool to drill a hole into the upper shin of the patient and insert the catheter directly into the bone marrow. As soon as he placed the IO and gave the medications, the patient's combativeness stopped.

"We basically watch this patient stop moving, slow down, and then they're fully paralyzed, and then he intubates," Annemarie said. With the airway secure, Sparrow then connected the patient to the portable ventilator that he carries in his gear.

When the roads finally cleared, Sparrow and the two paramedics were able to deliver the patient to the hospital fully stabilized. "It's a pretty massive undertaking outside of a hospital," Annemarie said. "We got that patient to the hospital, handed them off, and then—boom!—you can just go right to the ER. Their care [had] already started prior to them coming into the hospital."

The patient they rescued that snowy day is still going strong. "This is a really small place, and I don't want to give any patient identifiers," Annemarie told me, "but I knew this person. I knew their family. It's hard when these things happen in these small communities. I still see this individual around town, and that's all I think about. They have no recollection. They don't know who I am, but I know who they are. It's pretty amazing when you live in a small place where the impacts are felt immediately and long-lasting."

And without Sparrow's involvement? "I believe this patient probably would have died," she said.

Since then, Annemarie has had many similar experiences working with Sparrow. She told me that he's a crucial part of the team, and that he elevates her work and that of her fellow paramedics. "He brings you into the fold and gives you the courage through explanation and understanding to get your hands dirty . . . [to] get in there, do what needs to happen and support him while he's doing it."

This, she said, has led to a subtle but powerful shift in the role paramedics can play. "BC Ambulance has a mandate, you know? We don't stick around too long," she explained. "If [a call is] critical, then we do what we need to do, get in the ambulance and go. But Nic gives us this beautiful opportunity to 'stay and play,' if you will. This is the language that he likes to use . . . We're sticking around because there are a few interventions that we can do that are desperately needed in these moments. We're not delaying. We're just doing what's best for this patient, and then we're going to move."

What makes those interventions possible is Sparrow and his Tahoe full of life-saving equipment. An ER on wheels.

"We're trying to get [patients] to the hospital," Annemarie said. "But the hospital is here, right now. There's a physician here who's trained in these emergency or roadside procedures [and] he can do these massive interventions. So he's essentially buying time—not just for us but for these patients."

Sparrow has spent a decade trying to make EMS physicians like him the norm instead of the exception. To him, it makes perfect sense in rural and remote parts of Canada like the Kootenays to have doctors who can leave their hospitals or clinics and provide care in the field. "It brings resiliency to the country, having physicians who can . . . operate alongside paramedics and work with them as a team," he told me. "I think it's a very smart contingency plan for the country."

But Sparrow has had to swim upstream against powerful bureaucratic and cultural currents. For example, there was a time when he wasn't permitted to use lights and sirens when answering calls.

"In fact, we had the [fully equipped Tahoe] actually sitting on my driveway for about eight months before we got through the red tape," he said. "I have to admit I was quite angry about that particular situation, because we were responding to some very critical calls during those times. Even though we had met the criteria to be able to respond with lights and sirens, there's sometimes a lot of red tape to get through."

Then there were funding issues. As a registered charity, KERPA is fully funded by donations from individuals and businesses. It receives no money from the province, although some medications used in advanced life support, such as epinephrine, atropine and amiodarone, are provided. Everything else is purchased by KERPA through the charity, but even then, there are challenges. "Interestingly, because we're not a government agency, we're not allowed to use the same distribution centre as fire departments or search and rescue," Sparrow told me. "So we can't get discounts on equipment and stuff like that."

By now, he's used to obstacles being put in his way. "It's subtle things like that which make it difficult when maybe it doesn't have to be that way," he said. "But it's okay. We keep going . . . We're just going to keep going because we're trying to put patients first."

What's most surprising is that in the decade of KERPA's existence, Sparrow has never been paid to run the organization or respond to emergency calls. "I don't get paid anything. I don't bill MSP," he said, referring to BC's Medical Services Plan, the funding envelope for doctors. Until recently, his part-time emergency gig at Kootenay Lake Hospital helped support his family, including his six kids. But he quit the ER entirely so he could devote even more time to making KERPA a success. His wife works as a teacher, so there's that. It's a noble choice but a risky one.

Paramedics like Annemarie who have worked alongside Sparrow idolize him. But that's not the view generally held by paramedics in BC. Dr. Michael Christian knows a lot about that. Christian is a critical care specialist who, like Sparrow, has developed expertise in bringing critical care out into the field. A former paramedic, Christian served as the chief medical officer at BC Emergency Health Services from 2021 until early 2024. BCEHS runs the BC Ambulance Service.

"To be candid, I spent two years trying to stop the union from shutting him down when I was in that role," Christian told me. He was referring to the Ambulance Paramedics of BC, or APBC, which represents over 4,500 ambulance paramedics and emergency dispatchers in the province.

"There was a lot of pressure put on the leadership at BCEHS to not support Nic," Christian revealed, "to try to prevent him from doing what he was doing through different means." For instance, he said, APBC tried "to pressure the leadership [of BCEHS] to not sign the collaboration agreements they had with Nic." BC's Emergency Health Services Act restricts entities like KERPA from operating unless they sign collaboration agreements with the provincial health minister or BCEHS.

Some union members saw KERPA as a potential threat to their livelihood. "There's a significant degree of protectionism," Christian said. "The union here is strong. It's also unique because it represents one of the only remaining fully provincial services. So it's sort of one big body—a sort of David and Goliath—against Nic."

Sparrow is reluctant to talk about his difficulties in working with the union. "I can't speak for the paramedics as a whole," he told me. "I can only speak to some of the public comments we've had on our Facebook. 'You're not a professional organization. You're taking jobs away from paramedics. You're stopping advanced life support or critical care in the region. You'll never be able to respond. Physicians don't make a difference.' Those kinds of things."

Sparrow has fought those objections by hearing people out, by supporting paramedicine, both publicly and privately, and by providing training programs for paramedics through KERPA.

"Nic does a lot of work with these teams to help them with their skill sets," said Annemarie. "He does an amazing amount of liaising and training and partnership with these agencies. A lot of people understand what he brings when he comes to these scenes and are pretty grateful when that extra vehicle pulls up."

There is growing evidence that Sparrow's approach is the future. Mike Christian and several colleagues published a paper in 2024 showing that taking doctors like Sparrow out of the ER and putting them in the field saves lives. "I think that the tide is definitely changing," he told me. "I think he's pointing the way to the future. He's an innovator ahead of his time, and hopefully we're catching up to him."

This kind of feedback is music to the ears of Dr. Nic Sparrow.

"It has been hard, but anything worth pursuing is hard," he noted. "At the end of the day, come and live in our community and tell me that having an additional physician responding to these critical incidents isn't important. It totally is."

As Sparrow and I drove along the Crowsnest Highway linking Nelson and Castlegar, I thought about how he'd traversed these roads to rescue or ruin more than a thousand times. For most people, the highways of southeastern BC are conveyances and scenic routes, but for Sparrow, every twist and turn tells a story.

"What happened here?" I asked him.

"Two vehicles went head-on," he said. "The driver was trapped in [one] vehicle with bilateral broken femurs, which is a serious injury." He is right about that. When you break one thigh bone, never mind two, you can bleed to death. "This is a major trauma with potential for blood loss. KERPA was able to respond alongside paramedic crews and fire and police." Fortunately, the patient did not have life-threatening injuries to the airway, chest or abdomen. But that doesn't mean she wasn't in danger. "She was definitely shocked," Sparrow recalled.

He was able to help stanch the bleeding into the broken thigh bones by giving the patient tranexamic acid, or TXA, the blood-clotting medication I had used with Molly. He also gave the patient ketamine for pain and some midazolam to sedate her, got her on a monitor and then worked with the pre-hospital team on scene to extricate her from the vehicle. A chopper was dispatched to transport the patient to the closest trauma unit.

Sparrow told me that he's heard through the small-town grapevine that the patient is doing well. By his informal reckoning, that's the outcome for roughly nine out of every ten people he and KERPA attend to. But one in ten isn't so lucky. For those patients, and for Sparrow, it's a highway of tears. "I've talked with a number of families who have lost their kids," he told me. "When I say kids, it doesn't matter what age—twenty- and twenty-two-year-olds are still your kids."

For a moment, he appeared lost in thought. He stared out the windshield as if he was too emotional to make eye contact with me. "It's a highway of sorrow but [it] ends in hope," he said finally. "Literally, it ends in Hope, BC."

Sparrow seems to have plenty of hope. Hope that more people can be rescued. Hope that KERPA gets a permanent place in the healthcare landscape in BC and the rest of Canada. Hope that the organization can expand beyond just him.

He's forty-seven years old. Physically, he figures he can do this for another eight or ten years at most. "We're going to train other people behind me," he vowed, noting that KERPA was about to take on a second physician, and this person had already completed more than 260 hours of training, all of it unpaid. Sparrow is determined to have KERPA outlast him.

And if it doesn't?

"If no other physicians want to step up and do it and it's not adopted, then it's still not going to be in vain," he said. "We've helped a lot of people."

In my forty-plus years of emergency medicine, I've met lots of hardworking colleagues. Most of them complain about the system, and with good reason. Sparrow tries to build a better system. He may not succeed, but his attempt is noble. And I share his hope.

CHAPTER TEN

NO STONE UNTURNED

3:15 a.m.

Brian, can you reassess Hiromi?" Kosala sounds a bit concerned. Kosala is an experienced nurse who, like me, works mainly at night.

"Of course I can," I reply. "Who's Hiromi?" I've probably had that exact exchange with a nurse thousands of times during my career.

Before you start thinking bad thoughts about my memory or sense of caring, you should know that there are several plausible reasons why I don't recognize Hiromi's name. The first is that she might not be my patient. The emergency record may list me as the ER physician, but it's possible the patient was picked up by a colleague. Perhaps the actual physician in charge went home and forgot to hand Hiromi over to me or Samir, the night shift doctor.

It's also possible that Hiromi is a patient I've seen. It's just that I remember her not by her name but by her actual or suspected diagnosis. For many ER nurses, the main identifier is the patient's name; for ER doctors, what stands out is the patient's condition.

This time, however, it's none of the above.

"Hiromi is Ahu's patient," Kosala says.

"The woman with the kidney stone!" The tumblers click into

place. Hiromi is the patient Ahu mentioned to me just before she left in the ambulance with Britany. "What's up?"

"It's been hours and we're still waiting for her CT scan," says Kosala. "She started shaking, so I took her temperature. She's febrile."

"How high?" I ask.

"Thirty-nine point one."

"I'm coming," I reply.

I rush to a cubicle in the rapid assessment zone. Hiromi is holding the right side of her mid-back. That's not surprising, assuming that she does have a kidney stone. We call them kidney stones because they originate in the kidney, but the stone, a collection of minerals and salts often made of calcium, only causes pain once it moves into the ureter, a long, slender tube that drips urine made by the kidney into the bladder. A stone in the ureter blocks the flow of urine, and that causes urine to back up into the kidney, which causes intense pain.

Over my long career, most of the patients I've seen with kidney stones have extremely severe pain that begins suddenly, typically in the flank, and radiates to the abdomen or groin. The pain is a dull and constant ache with crescendos of cramping plus nausea and vomiting that make the experience almost unbearable.

Patients with appendicitis experience something similar except they tend to lie perfectly still because the inflamed appendix causes the peritoneum, or belly cavity, to also become inflamed. As a consequence, when you have appendicitis, every slight movement—even a tiny cough—produces sharp stabs of belly pain. Kidney stones are not like that because the swollen kidney sits behind the belly cavity and not in it. Thus, patients with kidney stones move about freely because movement does not cause pain. If anything, they pace around the room, sighing and moaning as they try in vain to find a comfortable position.

That Hiromi isn't pacing worries me a lot. She's as uncomfortable as any patient with a kidney stone. That she's holding her right flank tells me the stone is blocking the right kidney. But she's also sick with a high fever. She looks like she's too ill to writhe about.

"What's her blood pressure?" I ask Kosala as he adjusts her IV.

"One-fifteen over seventy," the nurse replies.

"Hiromi, that's the first bit of good news I've heard since coming to see you," I say to the patient. "I'm Dr. Goldman. My resident, Ahu, told me about you. You're obviously in pain. Have we given you something to make you more comfortable?"

"She got IV ketorolac two hours ago," Kosala confirms. "It seemed to hold her for a while, but the pain got much worse around the time she spiked a fever."

Ketorolac is an injectable anti-inflammatory medication we give to patients in severe pain. It's almost as effective as an opioid, with no risk of addiction.

"First things first," I tell Hiromi. "Let's give you something more to get the pain under better control."

"Morphine or hydromorphone?" asks Kosala.

"IV hydromorphone one to two milligrams every three hours as needed," I say. "And let's give her a litre of Ringer's lactate IV." This intravenous fluid replaces lost electrolytes in patients with low blood pressure.

"I'll get that ready now," he says as he leaves the cubicle.

"What did the doctors at the other hospital tell you?" I ask Hiromi. Ahu said she had visited another ER five days ago.

"They said I probably had a stone on the right side," she tells me.

"Did they do a CT scan?"

"They ordered one and I waited for hours, but it didn't happen," she says. "I felt better after they gave me something for the pain, and I just wanted to go home."

That happens all the time. The pain from kidney stones waxes and wanes. Between severe bouts, many patients feel fine. I've had lots of people who come to the ER with pain severe enough for me to order a CT scan, but if the pain subsides, they sometimes insist on going home rather than waiting for the scan.

"Did they make any arrangements to deal with the stone?"

"They gave me the phone number for the urology clinic and told me to make an appointment if the pain came back, which it did," she says. "I've left a couple of messages, but they haven't gotten back to me."

That's not surprising. There aren't enough urologists—the surgical specialists who deal with problems in the urinary tract, including kidney stones—and they tend to be extremely busy these days.

I pull out my pocket ultrasound probe and connect it to my phone. "This isn't a CT, but it will show me if you have a swollen kidney, which is what I'd expect to see if you have a big kidney stone," I tell her as I squeeze a dollop of ultrasound gel on my probe.

I place the probe near the back of Hiromi's right armpit. Watching the screen on my phone, I inch the probe until I identify the kidney sitting next to the back wall of the liver. Centring the kidney in the middle of the screen, I angle the probe gradually until what looks like a bear's paw pops into view. Radiologists use the term "bear's paw" to describe a kidney so swollen and dilated with urine that the swollen bits look like big, fat bear toes.

"Hiromi, your kidney is very swollen," I tell her. "I now have good reason to believe that you have a kidney stone, and that the stone is infected. That means infected urine is backing up from the stone into your kidney, and the infection has caused you to have a high fever. I'm going to start intravenous antibiotics, which will help. But we must find out where the stone is and either take it out or create a detour around it so we can drain off the infected urine instead of having it continue to back up. I'm going to start working on that right now."

Hiromi looks at me with fear in her eyes. "Was it a mistake to leave the other ER?"

When I was a much younger physician, I used to indulge myself by playing the "If only" game. If only the patient hadn't left against medical advice. If only the patient had come to the ER sooner. If only they had come to our hospital instead of "that other hospital." But I understand now that those musings are inherently self-aggrandizing. They're meant to make us feel our judgment is better than it is.

"I wasn't there when you decided to go home," I reply. "For you, it was the right thing to do at that moment. CT scans don't always happen when they're supposed to. Did you have a fever when you went to the first ER?"

"I had pain but no fever," she says.

"Then you had little reason to stick around when it was taking too long to get the CT," I reply. "All that matters is that you have a fever now and we need to deal with it."

I head back to the nursing station and pull up Hiromi's records from the other hospital.

"Locating, page urology stat," I ask the hospital switchboard operator. Hiromi's urine sample at the other hospital contained red blood cells, a telltale sign of a kidney stone. The urine sample did not contain white blood cells, which, if present, might indicate an infection.

Still, I can't help but wish Hiromi had waited around to get the CT scan. I'm concerned that she might have sepsis. Had the other hospital confirmed a large kidney stone and its precise location, it would have made my job saving her life easier and quicker.

"I've gotten blood and urine cultures and a serum lactate," Kosala tells me as he joins me at the nursing station.

Lactate is a chemical the body naturally produces when it's under stress. An elevated serum lactate level is commonly seen in patients with sepsis. Kosala is on the ball and has figured out what I'm thinking. He's also obtained blood and urine cultures, which detect infections, because these need to be taken before starting

IV antibiotics. If you collect cultures after starting the antibiotic, there's a good chance that the antibiotic will render the cultures negative, and you won't know which bacterium is causing the infection. Kosala has correctly anticipated that I'm going to start antibiotics now.

"Give Hiromi IV piperacillin four grams and tazobactam zero point five grams," I say. This is a powerful combination antibiotic for patients with sepsis due to a suspected kidney infection.

"What did your bedside ultrasound show?" he asks.

"Hiromi has a massively dilated kidney," I tell him. "The probable cause is a kidney stone. But we won't know much about the stone until we get the CT scan."

"Brian, urology on line two," says Vivica on the overhead speaker.

"Thanks for calling back so quickly," I tell the urology resident.

Kosala watches as I fill the specialist in on Hiromi's status and frantically scribble some notes.

"Urology won't be coming for at least three hours," I tell him as I hang up the phone. "They're about to do a kidney transplant."

Middle-of-the-night kidney transplants are not as unusual as you may think. The vast majority of transplanted kidneys come from deceased donors. The diagnosis of brain death and decisions around potential multiorgan donors are usually made during office hours. Donor kidneys are put on ice to slow down their degradation after they are removed from a body, and because donor organs can't stay on ice forever, kidney and other donor organ surgery is often done during the evening or at night.

Even if the urologist were available to see Hiromi immediately, they can't just go in and take out the stone without knowing precisely where it is, how big it is and how jagged it is. There's no way around it: Hiromi needs that CT scan ASAP.

"Locating, call the radiologist stat," I tell the switchboard operator.

It takes another five minutes, but the radiology resident calls back.

"I'm really sorry for the delay," the resident tells me on the phone. "One of the CT techs called in sick and we're short. And we had a couple of really challenging scans that took up a lot of the technicians' time. We should be able to clear the backlog shortly."

My conversation with the radiology resident reminds me that our overstretched healthcare system is precariously balanced on a knife's edge. Suddenly, I'm aware that I'm not the only physician with a patient in need of an emergency scan. I find it hard sometimes to declare that my patient is the sickest of the lot and needs to go first.

I just hope Hiromi remains stable.

We ER doctors and nurses are quick to complain when it's taking too long for our patients to get CT scans, ultrasounds and MRIs. We often fail to appreciate that we're missing half the story.

Jennifer Carey is a veteran medical radiation technologist, or MRT. That's the preferred title for the people who obtain X-rays, CTs, ultrasounds, MRIs and other diagnostic images. She told me that on most night shifts, MRTs like her are bombarded with requests for scans. "You have to fit everybody in," she said. "You're not just serving one department."

The reality is that we have a crisis-level shortage of skilled MRTs, and that is having a profound effect on the already chaotic operations of the country's ERs.

There are two types of MRTs: radiographers and radiation therapists (RTs). Jennifer is a radiographer. She obtains those exquisite scans that ER physicians like me depend on to make and confirm diagnoses. RTs set up and carry out courses of radiotherapy recommended by oncologists to treat many forms of cancer. Both are vital health professionals we doctors seldom talk about and you seldom read about.

For years, Jennifer has worked for Horizon Health Network in Moncton, New Brunswick. Horizon is the largest regional health authority in New Brunswick and the second largest health authority in Atlantic Canada. It operates twelve hospitals and more than a hundred medical facilities, clinics and offices throughout the province. She's also the manager of national advocacy for the Canadian Association of Medical Radiation Technologists (CAMRT). In that role, she has become the outspoken public face of the organization's more than 12,000 members. Part of what she does is battle stereotypes and slang terms that some health professionals use to describe the work that MRTs do.

"A lot of people think we're button pushers—that you just kind of lay a patient on the table and push a button and everything gets done automatically," Jennifer told me, sharing an ironic joke among MRTs that is based on an ill-informed view held by some doctors. "It looks easy because we're so good at our jobs. But it requires a lot of knowledge around the anatomy of the body, and how that anatomy changes when you move around the body, how that anatomy changes when it is diseased, sick or broken."

You can feel the pride MRTs have about their craft in good times. But now, post-Covid, they're under extraordinary pressure. "The amount of burnout the profession is experiencing is pretty profound," she said. "I think this applies to a lot of healthcare workers . . . It's part of our culture to kind of push through the pain. If you've got a really busy day, you push through it. You choose not to have your lunch because you just want to get through this next thing."

The "next thing" means another X-ray, CT or ultrasound. MRTs used to do three or four CT scans on a night shift, Jennifer told me, and have time for breaks. These days, it's ten times that on some nights. I'll explain how that happened in a bit, but the problem is a cavernous lack of MRTs exacerbated by record levels of absenteeism brought on by burnout and exhaustion. According to Jennifer, most hospitals are short MRTs every day.

"Vacancy rates have exponentially increased, and in some cases tripled across time within medical imaging and radiation therapy," wrote Laura Zychla and Mark Given in a 2024 article they co-authored on behalf of CAMRT and published in the *Journal of Medical Imaging and Radiation Sciences*. Zychla and Given show that in some imaging disciplines, such as ultrasound and mammography screening, the vacancy rates are in the double digits. The overall healthcare industry vacancy rate is half that, at 5.8 per cent, but even that, they noted, "is considered a crisis."

Those record-breaking levels of MRT absenteeism have an immediate impact on the increasingly swift flow of patients through the ER and the inpatient wards. Fewer MRTs means slower turnaround times for CT scans. It also means higher levels of stress for the MRTs who are still on the job. "Over the night shift, you're by yourself," Jennifer explained. "The phone's ringing . . . and they keep sending patients over . . . one right after another." MRTs who work nights have to quickly learn how to troubleshoot, she noted, "and you have to adapt and do a lot of the work yourself."

Being alone with a patient in the CT room brings its own challenges. For instance, every patient, regardless of illness, injury, body habitus (the general shape and build of a person's body, encompassing their physique, posture and body proportions) or demeanour, must be helped on and off the CT table. "We have roller boards to kind of help roll people onto the table," she explained. "If you're lucky enough, the porter who brought them over can stay to help you move the patient. But it's not the team of people that you might have on a day shift."

Like the rest of us, Jennifer has lots of war stories. She told me about one patient who'd been sent for a CT of the head and was thought to be under the influence of some kind of drug. She said it's not unusual for the ER to send over intoxicated patients in a state of stupor, but most wake up rather quickly, albeit in an agitated and disoriented state, the moment they're placed on the cold and unpadded CT table. "We have a joke in CT," she said, "that when they come over from trauma, we're either going to kill them or raise them from the dead."

This particular patient didn't respond when Jennifer spoke to him but was breathing on his own. The moment Jennifer helped him onto the CT table, he sat right up and was "pawing the air and very confused. And I'm trying to make it so that he doesn't fall off the table and so that he doesn't swat me in the head."

Fortunately for Jennifer, the porter who'd ferried the intoxicated patient to the CT room stayed around to help her control him. This is a scene that those of us who work in the ER, where there's always a team of people around, may have trouble picturing. In the end, Jennifer was able to complete the scan after calming down the patient.

Sometimes, the issue is far more grave than an angry or confused outburst. It's not unheard of, for example, for patients to suffer cardiac arrest right in the CT room. The sickest patients in the ER are usually the most likely to need urgent CTs, so it's not surprising that code blues sometimes happen there. When a patient codes in the ER, there's a team of healthcare providers right there with defined roles to play in the resuscitation efforts. Not so when someone has a cardiac arrest on the CT table.

Jennifer told me about one patient who needed a CT scan for a suspected aortic dissection. That's the same life-threatening condition affecting Britany, the young woman Ahu had accompanied to another hospital for emergency surgery. Unlike Britany, most people who have aortic dissections are older—Jennifer's patient was in her eighties—and have a history of high blood pressure, which puts stress on the aorta. Some aortic dissections, like Britany's, can be repaired surgically, while others are left untouched. The decision to fix the dissection is based on its location, its size and the age and overall health of the patient.

"She had a big aortic dissection," Jennifer recalled. "Big enough that they decided not to do anything with it because she was too old, and they figured that the surgery was going to be too much" for her to survive. But Jennifer didn't know any of this as she set up to do the scan. She was never told explicitly that the woman's dissection was not going to be repaired. The patient's doctor had ordered the scan not to plan for surgery but to keep an eye on the dissection.

So the woman was brought on a stretcher to the CT room to have the scan, but while she was being transferred from the stretcher onto the table, she had a cardiac arrest. Jennifer said instinct commanded her to jump in and start doing CPR. But not only was this not happening in a fully equipped resuscitation room in the ER, the patient wasn't even in the right position to do CPR. In the critical moments immediately after the woman's heart stopped, Jennifer was trying to lower the CT table so she could get her off and back onto the stretcher. She was also trying to learn whether the patient had a do-not-resuscitate (DNR) order on her chart, which would obviate the need to start CPR and summon the code blue team. And she was aware that the woman's two granddaughters were outside the door of the CT room and could likely hear the commotion going on.

Finally, Jennifer managed to yell to a colleague, who summoned the code blue team. They quickly came rushing in along with one of the ER physicians. The doctor talked to the granddaughters and also told Jennifer that the woman's aorta had probably burst spontaneously, which is the expected outcome of a large dissection that is not repaired. The code blue team also learned that the patient had a DNR order, and at that point, they terminated efforts to resuscitate the woman. She was pronounced dead on the stretcher in the radiology department.

"We were left shaking with that one," Jennifer told me. She remembers that story like it happened yesterday. But that wasn't her only time calling a code blue.

She told me about another incident involving a man who came to the ER with a gastrointestinal bleed and was sent to her for a CT scan. "This one was weird for me because he got up off the stretcher for some of his imaging and lay down," Jennifer said. Shortly after she finished the scan, the patient got back onto the stretcher and positioned himself on it with his legs over the side, saying, "I just need a minute."

"And he just hung his head," she recalled. "I waited a little bit, and he just didn't give any response." She checked his pulse and realized his heart had stopped. She pushed the button to call the code blue team, but until they got there, it was all up to her. This was actually her first cardiac arrest as a radiographer, and she said her adrenaline kicked in.

"It was instinct," she said. "You just kind of start doing the steps you have to do. The code team came and took over. I remember my legs were visibly shaking, and I had no control over them because of the adrenaline that was running through my body."

Unfortunately, the patient was not successfully resuscitated.

"I started to cry," Jennifer told me. "It wasn't just because I was sad for the patient. It's just your body being overwhelmed with whatever was happening that as soon as my part in that ended, my body just freaked out."

Later that day, one of the emergency physicians came around to explain that the patient had been feeling unwell for several days before coming to the ER. The cardiac arrest was likely due to profound blood loss from the gastrointestinal bleeding. Jennifer said the follow-up helped her process what had happened. But that kind of contact with an ER physician is unusual. She told me that she seldom feels part of the resuscitation team. And while it's routine nowadays for those teams to hold formal debriefing sessions after incidents to learn and share lessons, MRTs are rarely invited to participate.

"Often we are [viewed as] an accessory to the patient journey," she said. "When a patient goes south in the CT room, it's not necessarily front of mind to say we need to be included in debrief situations."

Incidents like these and other stressors have taken a huge personal toll on MRTs. My sense is that healthcare is increasingly recognizing the mental health toll on nurses, paramedics and other frontline providers. I'm less certain that the veil has been lifted on the sufferings of MRTs. "I think people are burnt-out," Jennifer told me. "Physically and mentally, they cannot do it anymore. They're pushed to the breaking point."

It wasn't always this way. MRTs used to love coming to work. Just ask Leslie MacLennan. She's seventeen years into a career as a radiation therapist at a hospital in Saint John, New Brunswick.

Radiation therapists operate linear accelerators and other machines to deliver a prescribed dose of radiation to shrink and in many cases eliminate cancers. Leslie described her RT training program as in some ways similar to a nursing degree and in some ways different. "It not just nursing and it's not just science," she told me. "It's this interesting mix . . . You really have to be heavy with the science and the technology. Our field is constantly advancing. The difference between when I started and today is like night and day. You have to be able to constantly adapt to it. We like learning about the evolving technology."

Leslie loves the physics part of the job. But she also loves the people part.

"I love the time that we spend with the patients," she told me. "I love meeting so many different people and learning their stories. When I was a student, one of the first things that pulled me to [RT] was this mix of nursing and science and human connection."

A big part of building that connection involves allaying the fears that patients bring to the clinic.

"Pretty much all of our patients are absolutely terrified," said Leslie. "When the machine is making its noise, there's a reason I'm hiding behind a concrete wall two doors away. We have to explain that to patients and [help them understand] why and how it's safe for them to receive this every day. We also have to explain how it is that we can get [to within] one millimetre of accuracy with a beam that they can't even see."

Leslie learned by working as part of a team that the key is to establish a personal connection with her patients. The team she started on at the beginning of her career had four members: a senior therapist who functioned as team leader, two experienced therapists and Leslie as the junior therapist. "When I first started, a lot of what they would get the younger therapists to do is to talk to the patients," she explained. "You bring them in, you ask them about their day, you learn about their stories, and you learn how they're experiencing cancer and help guide them through the side effects."

She said that in those days, some of the older machines were so primitive they required lots of time to calibrate. That had an unexpected benefit: More time calibrating the machines meant more time spent with patients, and more time to establish personal connections.

During her first year as an RT, Leslie worked with a mother of young kids whose breast cancer had metastasized to her brain. Leslie and her team administered a full course of palliative radiation to the woman's brain. The purpose of the radiation was not to eliminate the woman's cancer but to give her the best possible quality of life in the time she had left.

"It was right around Christmastime," Leslie recalled. "On paper, that would come across as quite sad. But instead, we had a wonderful week before Christmas. She was making special Christmas ornaments that her kids would have for their entire lives. We were spitballing ideas for Christmas stories she could write for them to take into next year [and beyond]. We really connected on that level, and she made a Christmas ornament for me, which I still have. I will never forget her, and I'll never forget that we were able to find joy even in what should have been a very, very sad time."

In effect, Leslie was learning to appreciate the value of applied empathy as she mastered applied physics. "It's not so much written in the textbook, but it is taught by the instructors to use your skills of active listening . . . It's the environment that we try to create in the clinic."

But that was then. Today, radiation therapy is more about clock-watching and less about empathy. Those forty-five-minute appointments have been scaled back to fifteen minutes or less.

"There has been a shift in how we speak with patients," Leslie told me. "It used to be that I would bring them into the room and have this casual chat before they even sat down on the bed. Now it's more walking and talking as we're going down the hall. Everything is more rushed."

Why did everything get so rushed? There are several reasons. An aging population means many more patients with cancer, and that means a greater demand for CTs, MRIs and ultrasounds. At the same time, diagnoses and treatment protocols are more complex than ever. Paradoxically, we have longer survival rates from cancer to thank for that. The patient with breast or lung cancer who would have lived two or three years in the past is now surviving nine or ten years or more. Those extra years are bought and paid for with extra diagnostic imaging and palliative radiation.

Then there's the lack of MRTs—an issue that CAMRT says has been decades in the making. A generation ago, a lack of radiographers and radiation technologists led some provinces to poach from others. There was also a big push to recruit new grads from other countries such as Australia.

When Leslie MacLennan was studying to be an RT nearly two decades ago, the shortage of technologists in New Brunswick was so profound that the province was sending patients to Maine to have radiation therapy. The province solved its shortage by hiring an entire graduating class from Quebec. "We were able to fully staff our machines," she explained. "The wait list dropped to zero, and it stayed there over the past twelve years. Then it started to creep up again."

So how do you squeeze more patients into the schedule without hiring more MRTs? By making the machines much more efficient. A scan of the chest or abdomen that once took thirty minutes or more can now be completed in just seconds. That technological marvel is good for patients and—at least in theory—good for the ER. But it's not good for already overworked MRTs.

"Over the past decade, CT and MRI exams have increased by thirty-six per cent and forty-six per cent, respectively," said Jennifer Carey. "But the number of MRTs has basically stayed the same. There hasn't been that investment in health human resource infrastructure." That means existing MRTs must work harder and more efficiently. If, for example, there is greater demand and longer waits for CTs and MRIs in the late afternoon and early evening, managers take radiographers off the day schedule and make them work evenings. "But they're not really adding any new positions to deal with the larger influx of demand," Jennifer noted.

RTs face similar issues, with one notable difference: There are limits on how much faster they can work the radiation therapy machines. "They need maintenance," Leslie told me. "They're only good for so many hours before they have to be replaced, and they cost $5 million to replace, so we have to be careful."

Basically, radiographers crank out CTs and MRIs faster than RTs can deliver radiation therapy. That means RTs feel like they are always under pressure to catch up. "Everything is an emergency," Leslie said. In the Saint John area, where she works, there may be seventy-five patients or more waiting for life-prolonging radiation therapy. Local oncologists, she told me, are always asking if she and her colleagues "could just work a little extra overtime." But they're already working overtime every day.

"There's a limited number of staff to run the machines and a limited number of hours in the day that we can run the machines," she explained. "There are no lunch breaks anymore. There are no coffee breaks anymore. We stagger and cover each other. Sometimes we come in on the weekends to try and get people through."

Meanwhile, MRTs have been retiring in droves. That cohort of skilled radiographers who arrived in Canada from Australia and filled depleted ranks years ago is now reaching retirement age. Until recently, colleges and universities in Canada were not enrolling enough students to replace them, and provinces weren't expanding service hours and locations. Then came Covid. The impact of the pandemic on nurses and physicians has been discussed at length, but its effect on MRTs was just as profound.

"That was a roller coaster of emotions, a roller coaster of policies, a roller coaster of procedure changes and a lot of fatigue during that process," Jennifer Carey told me. The pandemic put a virtual halt to non-urgent CTs and MRIs. "And then when Covid was over and things started to get back to normal, we had this backlog of all the people we couldn't image or treat now needing imaging."

The "solution" offered by hospitals and the provinces was to pack more CTs and MRIs into much longer days. That meant adding mandatory overtime to the already onerous burden on

MRTs. It also meant squeezing patients into shorter and shorter appointments.

"Like it or not, patients became a body part on the table that I have to image," said Jennifer. "Next one is a plain brain scan. Now we've got an abdomen and pelvis that we need to set up. We're pushing them through, and depersonalization starts to creep in. And that's one of the things leading to burnout."

Another contributor to burnout is the moral injury that RTs like Leslie feel when dozens of high-needs patients with cancer are waiting well beyond recommended guidelines for life-prolonging courses of radiation therapy.

Yes, there is a process. Oncologists rank their patients on a triage scale of one through four, with one being patients with the most immediate need. That includes, for example, patients with tumours compressing the spinal cord. Without immediate radiation, these patients are at risk of developing paraplegia or quadriplegia. Patients ranked fourth on the triage scale, on the other hand, have cancers that are slowly progressive, such as prostate cancer. Those patients can wait longer for radiation therapy. The moral injury comes from knowing that every patient waiting should not have to wait.

"It's rationing something that should be available for everybody as they need it," said Leslie. "There's some cutting of corners [or] whatever expression you want to use. You are hoping that [the fourth-ranked patients] are the least risky to wait, but it's rationing."

Leslie told me that this situation is personal for her. In 2017, at age thirty-three, she was diagnosed with breast cancer. She had a mastectomy, chemotherapy and radiation. "I started my radiation at a time when we didn't have a wait list," she said. "If I was in the exact same position today, in 2024, I would be waiting twelve weeks to start my radiation, when the benchmark is eight weeks. We even have patients waiting sixteen weeks."

Leslie can't help but empathize with them. "You're sitting at home just waiting to complete this chapter of a hellish year," she said, "and now you must wait three months to even start the final phase. When I put myself in their shoes, which we often do as therapists, it's just heartbreaking. You feel that stress; you feel that heartbreak."

As a radiographer, Jennifer Carey is shielded from the emotional repercussions of rationing radiation therapy, but her moral injury comes from watching the images as they're generated in the CT room.

"I think one thing that people don't fully understand is that we see what's wrong with a patient before anyone else does," she explained. "We see what is broken. We see the cancer that they don't know they have. We see the brain tumour that they don't know they have yet."

She told me about one four-year-old patient who was brought to the ER after having an epileptic seizure. The emergency physician ordered a CT scan, and the child was taken to Jennifer's department.

"When they are children," she said, "we let the parent into the CT room with a lead shield on"—to protect against radiation—"because it's comforting to the child to have the parent there." The way the room was set up, Jennifer knew the mother could see her eyes as the images appeared on the monitor. "I can feel her staring at me the entire time her child is in the scanner," she recalled, "because she is looking for whether or not my face will crack and give her an indication of whether or not her child is going to die."

Sadly, a cancer showed up on the view screen.

"As soon as that golf-ball-size tumour pops up in that child's brain stem, I know that this is going to change their lives forever," she said.

The child had a brain stem glioma. That's a type of tumour seen in kids that originates in the brain stem, which connects the two hemispheres of the brain to the spinal cord and cerebellum. There are two main types of gliomas in children, diffuse and focal. Diffuse brain stem gliomas are the more common. They tend to be high-grade tumours and are very aggressive. Diffuse brain stem gliomas are hard to remove and are usually treated with radiation therapy. Focal brain stem gliomas occur in one area or are contained within a small part of the brain stem. They tend to be benign, and they're easier to treat and have a better prognosis. Because they grow slowly, focal brain stem gliomas can be watched for a time and then surgically removed and treated with radiation therapy and chemo. Additional treatment may be needed if the tumour grows back.

Remember that Jennifer isn't an oncologist or an oncology nurse. Her job is to do CT scans. When she saw the tumour, her only job was to complete the scan and not think about the emotional implications of what she'd seen on her screen.

"I have to shut down whatever I see and whatever I'm feeling and go out there and pretend that nothing is wrong," she told me. "That happens every day. Maybe not as intense as the mother staring at me. But every day, we diagnose cancer for the first time. Every day, we diagnose a disease, or we check for metastases, or we check to see whether the cancer is shrinking or getting larger."

The emotional burden is so intense that every few months, Jennifer needs to take a break from doing CT or MRI scans to do something less intense, like taking X-rays to look for broken bones.

I've been an ER physician for more than four decades, and I've never thought as deeply about what it's like to do the work of an MRT as I'm doing on these pages right now. The interminable workload. The complexity. The gravity. The emotional burden. All of these things help explain why CT scans can't be produced with the speed and predictability of a pizza delivery.

"I can understand how people in the ER think the people doing CTs are slow tonight," Jennifer said. "What they don't know is that I have an ICU patient on the table, and the neuro ICU is calling with a patient who might have a brain bleed and needs a scan right now. I don't think different areas of the hospital understand how we work together and where delays can happen."

I do now. I'm sorry it has taken me to the last stages of my career in the ER to do so.

3:45 a.m.

I'm looking at Hiromi's CT scan when the radiology resident calls me on my cellphone. In the middle of the night, a radiologist will usually post a report to the radiology reporting software system, where I can read it at my leisure. When they call you, it's urgent.

"Have you seen the scan?" the resident asks.

My eyes widen as I click through the first few images. "The kidney looks really swollen," I reply.

"Very swollen and inflamed," says the resident. "If you scroll down about eight images, you will see a large, jagged stone in the proximal ureter."

"I see it."

"In my opinion, that stone is not going to pass without help."

"Thanks for letting me know," I say.

I walk quickly to Hiromi's bedside to check the last temperature taken. It's 38.6 Celsius. Kosala joins me in the cubicle.

"Hiromi's blood pressure is ninety-two over fifty-eight," he says. "I was going to let you know, but you beat me to it and came here on your own."

Hiromi's temperature is a bit lower since she received powerful intravenous antibiotics. But the fact that her blood pressure is going down makes me worry that she's succumbing to sepsis.

"What's her serum lactate level?" I ask the nurse.

"It's three point four millimoles per litre," Kosala replies.

That's ominous. A normal serum lactate level is up to one millimole per litre. 0.5–1 mmol/L. Hiromi's lactate level is in the range of moderate elevation. It's a level that confirms to me that Hiromi has sepsis. The risk of dying from sepsis caused by an infected kidney stone can be as high as an eye-popping 27.2 per cent. Antibiotics aren't enough to save lives. The stone must be removed by a urologist, and quickly.

"Hiromi, where's your family?" I ask her.

"My mother and my brother live in Vancouver," she says. "Is it that serious?"

"You have an infection in your bloodstream caused by the kidney stone," I tell her. "I think your family would want to know."

"Am I going to die?" The world always stops for me the moment a patient asks that question.

"You're young and strong and are otherwise healthy," I tell her as I give her hand a gentle squeeze. "You have most of the important things going for you."

As I turn and stride quickly out of Hiromi's room, I call the switchboard operator and ask her to page urology right away.

"They're still in the OR," the operator replies. "Shall I hold the call?"

I just remembered! The urology resident is doing a kidney transplant and won't be able to provide immediate assistance. My best guess is that the transplant will still take another three hours, assuming all goes well.

"Have them call me as soon as they're out of the OR," I reply.

"Kosala, tell Cynthia we have another customer for resus," I tell him as I get back on my phone. "Switchboard, page ICU."

The people who work in the intensive care unit do magnificent work keeping alive patients who are at the brink of death. But even their miracles won't save Hiromi unless we get that infection out of her kidney.

Kidney stones are incredibly common. In any given year, a whopping 2.1 per cent of the population has one. But infected kidney stones are much less common, and sepsis caused by an infected kidney stone is downright rare. So rare that for many of us, a patient with sepsis from an infected kidney stone is a once-in-a-career event. By dint of luck, I've seen a few of them.

In addition, I have a sideline testifying as an expert witness in medical malpractice cases involving ER physicians who've been sued for negligence by patients or surviving family members. As I think about Hiromi, one such case comes vividly to mind. The patient was a middle-aged woman who died of sepsis caused by an infected kidney stone. As part of my work as an expert witness, I read up on how to diagnose and treat infected stones in the ER. From that, I learned that there's another way to save the patient—one that does not require the services of a urologist.

3:55 a.m.

"Page the interventional radiologist stat," I tell the switchboard operator.

Interventional radiology, or IR, was born as a subspecialty of radiology more than six decades ago. The idea behind it is to use ultrasounds, X-rays and later CT scans to guide treatment and transform radiologists from makers of diagnostic images into treaters of diseases.

The first interventional procedure involved unblocking a leg artery in a woman with gangrene. The procedure saved the woman from a foot amputation. Since then, IR has exploded. Today, IR specialists insert semi-permanent catheters into the large central veins of patients with cancer or deep infections so that they can receive long-term medical therapies. They zap cancers with heat or high-dose chemo. They drip drugs into blocked arteries and veins to dissolve clots. They inject bone cement into fractured vertebrae to heal them. They shrink fibroids, which are tumours in the womb.

They also do a certain procedure that just might save Hiromi's life.

"Interventional radiology is on line two," says Vivica.

"Dr. Goldman here." I know I sound a bit winded. "I have a thirty-one-year-old woman with sepsis from an infected kidney stone. The stone is one point five centimetres at its widest diameter and jagged. The stone is lodged in the proximal ureter. The patient is febrile and hypotensive with an elevated lactate."

That's the background. Here comes the pitch.

"I need you to insert a nephrostomy tube proximal to the stone," I say. A nephrostomy tube is a thin, flexible catheter that an IR specialist inserts through the skin overlying a patient's ureter, which is located in the mid to upper back. The radiologist doesn't have the tools to remove the infected stone but does have the tech and the know-how to access and drain off the infected urine that's backing up behind it. And that may buy us enough time to get Hiromi's infection under control.

"Have you called urology?" asks the IR.

"They're doing a renal transplant and aren't available."

"I'll be there as soon as I can."

In the resuscitation room, Hiromi's blood pressure has dropped to 80 over 45. The ICU resident has started her on intravenous norepinephrine, a medication administered to patients in shock due to sepsis and other causes. The goal is to raise her blood pressure and buy time for the IR specialist to do the procedure.

4:20 a.m.

Hiromi is taken to the radiology department, where the IR specialist uses an ultrasound probe—like the one I carry—to locate the ureter. She disinfects and anesthesizes the skin on Hiromi's back, then carefully inserts a needle and syringe until the needle is inside the ureter. The syringe is removed and a guidewire threaded through the needle until it's also inside the ureter. The needle is then withdrawn, and a nephrostomy tube is carefully threaded over the guidewire. If all has gone well, cloudy—infected—urine starts to drip out of the tube. The nephrostomy tube is then sutured in place so it doesn't fall out. The tube is connected to a plastic bag taped to Hiromi's back so infected urine can be collected and measured.

After about twenty minutes, the IR phones me with the good news. "We got it," she says. "We got out forty millilitres of some really infected-looking pee."

"How's our patient doing?" I ask.

"Better," she says. "Her blood pressure is one-ten over seventy. The critical care doctors are taking her to the ICU. She was very sick."

"You got it done blindingly fast."

"I ran through several red lights to get here," she says.

"Thank you for saving Hiromi's life," I tell her.

"You're welcome," she says. "I've done a fair number of nephrostomy tubes at this stage of my career, but this is the first time I've done one where the immediate stakes were so high."

I walk across the ER to the rapid assessment zone to give Kosala the good news. A "slow night" in the CT room delayed Hiromi's diagnosis. But on this night, one fast-working specialist was the difference between life and death.

Vivica stops me as I walk by the main nursing station. "Dr. Goldman, I have Hiromi's mother on the line. She's calling from Vancouver."

It's a lot easier speaking with loved ones calling from faraway places when the prognosis flips from guarded to fair.

CHAPTER ELEVEN

SAVE ME

5:10 a.m.

Samir approaches me warily. "Brian, can I meet you at triage?" I have a hunch that I know why.

"You want me to stay!"

The grin on my face makes Samir relax. Some emergency physicians dislike asking for help dealing with the volume of sick and injured patients because they think it makes them look incapable of doing their jobs. An unprompted offer is much more likely to be received well.

"It's busy," says Samir. "I really appreciate it."

"It's much less of a bother than you think," I reply. "When you're the night doc, it's your responsibility to see every patient, at least in theory."

"At least in theory," replies Samir. He's half my age. That the two of us are in sync makes me feel young.

"Now that the two of you have bonded, do you mind seeing some patients in the waiting room?" Cynthia tries to sound bossy.

"I just picked up a patient in resus," says Samir, looking at me. "Do you mind helping thin the herd out here? Feel free to cherry-pick." He's giving me permission to choose patients who are easier to sort out and discharge without an extensive diagnostic workup and treatment.

At least in theory.

That exchange with Samir reminds me of the casual way ER physicians sacrifice a good night's sleep. On casino shifts, I seldom go home before four or five in the morning. As I near retirement, I find myself caring less and less about the sleep I'm missing.

In the same way, ER physicians don't care all that much about the evenings and weekends that we work. That includes long weekends. To me, a Saturday-evening shift is exactly like your Monday morning. Life-threatening illnesses and motor vehicle accidents don't take a holiday, so why should we.

It does mean that we sometimes miss family gatherings and other special occasions. And yes, we complain, sometimes bitterly. But being there in a patient's hour of need can be a reward far more profound than the fellowship of an important social occasion. Just ask Dr. Trevor Jain.

The ER physician and director of the Bachelor of Science in Paramedicine program at the University of Prince Edward Island has missed many a social gathering as an army reservist, serving as a trauma team physician and medical director in war zones such as Bosnia, Kuwait and Iraq.

There was that time when Jain missed his own birthday celebration. It happened during a blizzard. Snowstorms in rural PEI can shut down the island. It means patients cannot be transported to larger hospitals on the mainland. It means doctors like Jain and the nurse who work with him are on their own.

"We got an ambulance call that they were bringing in a teenager who was found on the side of the road in the blizzard," Jain recalled. The patient, a sixteen-year-old, had collapsed in a ditch while walking. It was minus fifteen degrees Celsius at the time. The teen was dressed in a T-shirt and jeans. The paramedics found him in full cardiac arrest. His body was so cold and stiff, the paramedics had difficulty doing CPR chest compressions. At first, the heart monitor showed no discernible rhythm. Twice en route to the hospital by ambulance, the teen went into ventricular fibrillation. Paramedics shocked the teen's heart but got no response.

It was 9:30 p.m. Jain was at the hospital but off duty and preparing to go home. "It was my birthday, and my family was waiting for me," he recalled. The physician on duty that evening did not feel comfortable trying to save the teen. She asked Jain to take the case.

"I was in my civvies . . . my jeans and my sweater," said Jain. "I didn't change back into scrubs."

From the dispatcher's report on the radio, it was obvious to Jain that the teen was suffering from hypothermia, a condition that occurs when the patient's body temperature drops below 35 degrees Celsius. Hypothermia is a medical emergency because it causes the heart, nervous system and other organs to shut down. The lower the temperature, the greater the chance of dying.

The teen had two things going for him. The first was his age. Infants and teens are more likely than older patients to survive a hypothermic cardiac arrest. The second was the cold itself. A lower body temperature slows down the body's metabolism. During that time, the brain and heart require less oxygen and will show less damage once resuscitated. In 2018, the journal *Annals of Emergency Medicine* published a case report of a thirty-one-year-old man who was rescued off a mountain in Italy. He was in cardiac arrest for nearly nine hours before being successfully resuscitated and made a full recovery.

Paramedics brought the team to the resuscitation room where Jain and the nurses were standing by. "He looked like he was dead," said Jain. "He was stiff to touch." Jain wondered if the teen had frozen to death.

Over my four-decade career, I've seen lots of patients with hypothermia, mostly unhoused people who arrive semi-conscious with a core temperature of 32 or 33 degrees Celsius. Treating them is a snap: warming blankets, heated IV fluids and heated humidified oxygen to breathe. This teen was totally different. A nurse hooked him up to a monitor to check his vital signs.

"The temperature was twenty-six," said Jain. "I was just shocked." He had never treated a patient with a temperature that low before. I'd have been shocked too.

To give the boy any chance at all at survival, Jain and the nurses had to warm his body up as fast as possible. Unfortunately, Jain and his colleagues didn't have at their disposal the fastest and most effective means of rewarming. It's called extracorporeal membrane oxygenation, or ECMO. It works by taking blood out of a patient's body, pumping it through a machine that acts like an artificial lung to add oxygen and remove carbon dioxide, then returning the oxygenated blood back into the body, essentially allowing the patient's heart and lungs to rest and recover when they are unable to function properly on their own. In the case of hypothermia, ECMO can also warm the blood before returning it to the body. ECMO has become the preferred treatment for hypothermic cardiac arrest because it can rewarm the body at a rate of up to ten degrees Celsius per hour. The survival rates with ECMO are as high as 47 per cent.

If Jain didn't have ECMO, he was determined to do his best to save the boy. "I said, 'Nurses, we're going to do something that we haven't done before,'" Jain recalled telling them. The technique he tried is called thoracic lavage, and it was first described in a case report in 1990. It involves placing four large-calibre tubes into the chest, two on each side between the second and third ribs in the front of the chest and another two on each side between the fifth and sixth ribs in the back, then infusing the chest cavity with warm sterile salt water. It's not as effective as ECMO, but it can raise the core temperature by three degrees Celsius per hour.

Jain and the nurses gathered supplies and machines to warm the fluid that would be infused into the teen's chest. "It was surreal," said Jain. "The trauma bay was noisy but oddly quiet at the same time. They talk about entering a state of flow. We had the right people working . . . some very senior nurses and they figured it out. They jury-rigged it to get the chest tubes all set up."

In addition to the chest tubes, Jain intubated the teen, and a respiratory therapist fed warm humidified oxygen through the ventilator. They also put a catheter into the teen's belly cavity to infuse warm fluids there.

Over the ensuing three hours, the teen's body temperature remained stubbornly low. Jain said they tried shocking his heart fourteen times over that period, to no effect. Jain and the team were starting to doubt the teen would survive. Then, his body temperature hit 29 degrees and his heart rhythm changed to one that was irregular. To Jain, it was a sign that the teen's heart was warming up. "He's going to make it," Jain recalled saying out loud.

When the teen's body temperature reached 31 degrees, they detected a normal heart rhythm and a strong pulse. The teen was admitted to the hospital's ICU, still intubated and on a ventilator, with the various chest and other tubes clamped off in case they were needed again.

By the next morning, the teen, still intubated, was conscious enough to be able to nod his head and squeeze his loved ones' hands. "I went and visited him in the ICU," said Jain, choking up as he told me. "He looked at me and I just said, 'I'm so glad you're here.' And he just looked at me with his eyes.'"

Jain says the teen's only lasting injury was second-degree frostbite on one of his shoulders. He walked out of the hospital alive and well. Today, he works in the commercial fishing industry and is married.

Jain told me he got home around two in the morning on the day following his birthday. "I just went upstairs and looked at my daughter, who was sleeping," he said. "I checked in on my wife and [then] I just sat in the sunroom and watched the snow coming down."

It wasn't the birthday present he'd been expecting. But it was the birthday present he needed. And you know what? It's the birthday present every ER physician would do almost anything to have.

"Brian!" A familiar voice makes me turn towards the waiting room. It's Ahu, and she has a giddy expression on her face.

"The prodigal resident returns!" I'm genuinely glad to see my protégé. "How did the transfer go? And how's Britany?"

"It was so awesome," she says. "Britany was stable most of the way, but just as we rounded the corner to pull in to emergency, her pain got worse. I checked her BP, and it was one twenty-five over eighty-five."

"What did you do?" I love hearing Ahu talk about her patients.

"I gave her twenty milligrams of labetalol IV, and her systolic BP dropped to one hundred," she says. "You know what? Her pain settled down! I couldn't believe it."

"And then what happened?"

"I handed Britany off to the fellow in cardiovascular surgery," she says. "When I mentioned the spike in her BP and how I responded, she said I did the right thing." Ahu is beaming. "I feel like a real physician. You learn about clinical findings, diagnosis and treatment, but they aren't real until you apply them to an actual patient in distress."

"I'm proud of you," I tell her. I remember moments like this from my own training days.

"I hear you saved Hiromi's life," says Ahu, changing the subject.

"To be perfectly correct, an interventional radiologist saved Hiromi's life," I reply.

"You're being modest," she says. "I was worried about her, but you made the diagnosis."

"And in the future, so will you."

"Okay, back to work," she says. "Can I talk to you about a patient I just saw in the waiting room?"

"Fire away."

"Theo is apparently a regular," she says. "He's a twenty-six-year-old guy with a history of fentanyl use disorder. He was found collapsed in an alleyway downtown. Bystanders called 911."

"Did he get naloxone?" I inquire. Naloxone is a medication that temporarily reverses the effects of an opioid drug like fentanyl. When I was in medical school, naloxone was used exclusively by frontline healthcare providers. In March 2016, Health Canada changed it to non-prescription. Since June 2016, in Ontario it has been available for free through pharmacies, community organizations and provincial correctional facilities. Other provinces followed suit at different times (for example, BC in September 2016, Alberta in February 2017 and Saskatchewan in April 2018).

Anyone can get naloxone kits and even some training in how to respond to an overdose.

The naloxone I was taught to give was administered as an intravenous dose. I can still remember the first time I gave it to a patient in the ER who had taken an overdose of heroin. He was unconscious and taking just six breaths a minute. His pupils were tiny, like periods at the end of a sentence. I pushed a dose of 0.4 milligrams of naloxone. Boom! Immediately, the guy was breathing faster and faster, taking big gulps of oxygen. His pupils got larger before my eyes. Then he woke up and looked around as if he'd just risen from the dead and wanted to see what he'd missed. That was the first time I felt like I'd saved a life.

"The paramedics found a spent dose of intranasal naloxone beside Theo," Ahu tells me, "along with drug paraphernalia."

"Let me guess—there were no witnesses."

"You're right."

Given how fast fentanyl gets into the system once injected, I knew it was unlikely that Theo had given himself a dose of naloxone. It was far more probable that someone who was with him saw that he'd overdosed, gave him naloxone to save his life and called 911 before leaving the scene.

Stuart McKinnon knows all about the impact of the opioid crisis. He's a veteran paramedic in Muskoka, a particularly bucolic part of Ontario's cottage country, east of Georgian Bay. More than 60,000 Ontarians live permanently in Muskoka in places like Huntsville, Gravenhurst and Bracebridge. Many thousands more flock to cottages there every summer.

The opioid epidemic may have started in Canada's cities, but rural areas haven't escaped it. McKinnon reckons that in Muskoka, opioid overdoses have doubled since 2018. It's a problem made worse by the geographic realities of living in a sparsely populated part of the province. "You can't always rely on a paramedic or a firefighter or the Ontario Provincial Police or a healthcare provider nearby," he told me.

McKinnon, who is the deputy chief of Muskoka Paramedic Services, thinks the way to save lives is to empower bystanders to help. That means distributing to the public kits with pre-loaded intranasal naloxone, gloves and a respirator. In 2023, Ontario made it mandatory to have these kits in high-risk workplaces such as construction sites. (The construction industry has been extremely hard hit by the opioid crisis.) The province considers a workplace to be high risk if someone has overdosed there in the past or if employees have seen co-workers using opioids. "It's all about making people comfortable using the kits because it saves lives," McKinnon said. "It's about getting them in [employees'] hands. It's educating people and having open, honest conversations about opioid use."

McKinnon told me about one 911 call he responded to years ago. "Somebody obviously made the phone call," he said. "When we arrived, there was a young person on the front porch of this home who had been involved in a [drug] poisoning. And we had no other information—nothing to go by. Somebody had left this individual to die. They tried their best by calling 911 but they fled the scene."

There are many reasons why bystanders leave the scene of an overdose. They might be afraid of being charged with possession or even trafficking of illegal substances. If the overdose victim dies, they might fear getting caught up in a criminal investigation. And in small towns, where everyone knows everyone else, there's often a fear of being recognized. "It's about stigma," McKinnon said.

Since 2017, Canada has had a law that provides some legal protections for people who seek emergency help during an overdose. The Good Samaritan Drug Overdose Act applies to anyone who seeks emergency support during an overdose, including the person experiencing the overdose. It shields bystanders who are in possession of controlled substances or have themselves consumed controlled substances. It also protects them from liability, whether they stay or leave the scene before help arrives.

These days, bystanders, first responders and ER physicians are doling out more naloxone than ever, but they seldom get thanks for it. While the miracle med delivers intoxicated patients from the jaws of death, it also puts the patient into severe opioid withdrawal, sometimes with disturbing consequences.

Dawn Gavin, the veteran triage nurse at the Queen Elizabeth II Health Sciences Centre in Halifax, told me one story about a patient who had overdosed and was unresponsive when he was brought into her ER. The doctor gave the patient a syringeful of

IV naloxone, and he promptly woke up, unhappy to be in opioid withdrawal. "He grabbed the uncapped syringe"—which the doctor had put on the bedside table—"and started to come at me," she told me. "There was a police officer that was there with another patient, and she intervened. He punched her in the face and broke her jaw. At the end of it, we had six police officers and tasers and guns out, trying to control this individual."

I'm thinking of that story as Ahu leads me down the hall of EMS stretchers to a very irritable young man in a threadbare sequined rainbow-coloured tuxedo jacket. He's standing up and leaning against a stretcher.

"Joseph, I haven't seen you in ages." I extend my fist for a bump, but the gesture is not reciprocated. "How have you been?"

"Stop being a jerk," the patient replies.

"I thought his name was Theo?" says Ahu, looking at the chart.

"We've called him Joseph since the first time he came in wearing his amazing technicolour dreamcoat."

"Hey, Doc, I feel like shit and I want to go," says Theo-Joseph with a great big yawn.

"Ahu, what's going on here?" I ask.

"He's supposed to be in withdrawal," she says. "But aside from being irritable and yawning, I'm not seeing it."

"Pay no attention to the lady, Doc," says Theo-Joseph. "I'm dope sick."

"When was your last hit of fentanyl?" I ask him.

"I don't remember."

"The paramedics say it happened just before 2 a.m. That's too soon to be dope sick," offers Ahu, using the same slang term for the symptoms of opiate withdrawal as the patient did.

For regular users of street fentanyl, withdrawal symptoms can start as soon as twelve hours after the most recent dose. There are drugs that can relieve those symptoms and the cravings for more opioids. Suboxone, for example, is a combination of naloxone and a second drug called buprenorphine and is administered as a pill that dissolves under the tongue. But it can't be given until at least twelve hours have passed. If it's given too early, it will hasten the arrival of withdrawal symptoms and decrease the likelihood that the patient will agree to continue taking Suboxone.

"You're going to have to stay here for several hours before we can give you medications to help with dope sickness," I tell him. "Have you taken Suboxone before?"

"I took it for several months last year," he says. "But I started using again."

"Relapses are common," I tell him. "Want to give it another try?"

"If you give it to me now, I'll take it," says Theo-Joseph.

Ahu interjects. "If you've taken Suboxone before, you know we can't start it here in the ER until you have moderate withdrawal symptoms."

We could give Theo-Joseph a prescription for Suboxone to start using at home in a few hours, but he has other ideas.

"Just give me some hydromorphone," he says.

"That won't help you," Ahu replies.

"Oh yes it will."

I'm betting that Theo-Joseph is anticipating how bad withdrawal can be. And it can be very bad. People describe it as a sickness so severe they feel like they're dying. It's the physical symptoms—sweats, nausea, severe aches and diarrhea—in combination with anxiety and depression that make it so unpleasant.

It's also knowing that temporary relief is just a puff of fentanyl or an IV hit of hydromorphone away.

"Hydromorphone would relieve your cravings temporarily," says Ahu. "But you'd have stronger cravings as soon as it wears off."

"We'd just be kicking the can down the road," I add. "Why don't you hop back up on the stretcher? We can give you IV fluids. We can give you something for your nausea and something for your antsy feeling."

"Okay, I'll stay," says Theo-Joseph.

"It'll get bumpy in a few hours," I acknowledge, "but we can help get you through this."

Ahu and I walk back towards the triage area.

"Do you think he'll stay?" she asks me.

"I honestly don't know."

The opioid crisis has left an enormous trail of accidental deaths and shattered family lives. Between 2016 and 2023, roughly 45,000 Canadians lost their lives to opioid poisonings, according to the federal government. Most of those were young men aged thirty to thirty-nine. In 2023, 82 per cent of those deaths involved fentanyl. That's an increase of 44 per cent since 2016.

The toll that the opioid crisis has taken on emergency medicine has been equally staggering. The government reports that between 2016 and 2023, 175,000 patients went to ERs across Canada to seek treatment for opioid-related poisonings. Fully 45 per cent of those poisonings involved fentanyl, and three-quarters were accidental. Like Theo-Joseph, the majority of those who were treated in the ER were men between the ages of twenty and forty-nine.

According to a study published in the journal *PLOS One*, opioid-related ER visits in Ontario increased by 165 per cent between 2009 and 2019, while the number of patients transported to hospital by paramedics jumped by a whopping 429 per cent. (Patients who are poisoned with fentanyl seldom walk into the ER on their own.) Those increases were not uniformly distributed. For instance, in the region that encompasses Hamilton, Niagara, Haldimand and Brant, in the southeastern part of the province, ER visits quadrupled from 500 to more than 2,200 over that same period, while paramedic transports to ERs increased sevenfold, from 217 to over 1,600.

The Greater Toronto Area happens to be one of the epicentres of the opioid overdose epidemic in Canada. Toronto Public Health (TPH) says that in 2023, there were 523 reported opioid toxicity deaths in the city. That's up slightly over 2022. TPH also reports that Toronto's paramedics were kept extremely busy. Between July 1, 2023, and June 30, 2024, there were 4,874 opioid-related calls for paramedics. The calls included both fatal and non-fatal opioid overdoses.

TPH says the highest concentration of calls for suspected opioid overdoses was in the downtown area. Dr. Kashif Pirzada undoubtedly took care of many of those patients. He's the ER physician we met earlier who works at two of the highest-volume ERs in the GTA.

Pirzada told me that he sees a lot of patients with fentanyl intoxication. Some are heavily sedated and require a lot of intervention. Others are quickly revived—so quickly that they often don't stay long enough to be assessed by physicians. "They'll get revived by naloxone," he explained, "and they leave half an hour later."

The ones who can't be discharged quickly can be hard to treat, adding to the already huge volume of patients Pirzada and his colleagues see. Some may need to be intubated and put on ventilators, he said. They often require time-consuming critical care. And like Joseph, they may end up in the ER over and over again.

Ideally, the goal is to help patients into recovery, but that can be both challenging and frustrating, especially in high-volume ERs like the ones where Pirzada works. "We have a Suboxone protocol," he told me. "We can start someone on Suboxone right there [in the ER]. I've had maybe one out of a hundred take it. When people are in the acute phase of addiction, the willingness is not there. Most will just decline what we offer them and leave."

For some overdose patients, the entrance to the ER may as well be a revolving door. "We're seeing some of them two, three, four, five times in a row," he told me. "They're in this pattern of overdosing recurrently over a few weeks. Trying to direct people out of the addiction life is hard. Their lives are extremely chaotic."

Pirzada says that when he and his colleagues see the same patients repeatedly in a short period of time, they wonder if there's more they can do. They have even explored the possibility of certifying them under provincial mental health legislation so they can be admitted involuntarily.

Compulsory treatment for addiction has become a hot political topic across Canada lately. With very few exceptions, in Western society it is a fundamental right of all human beings to refuse treatment, and that includes people who are incarcerated. There are very few historical exceptions to this basic tenet. They include treating patients with severe psychiatric diseases who are admitted to mental health facilities and treating incarcerated individuals with HIV and other communicable diseases.

The compulsory treatment of incarcerated individuals with addiction is a relatively recent addition to the list. On the one hand, one can argue that there is virtue in society's efforts to help people with severe addiction enter recovery. On the other hand, coercing those individuals to accept treatment as a condition of their sentencing violates their right to personal autonomy. As well, it is a bedrock principle that addiction treatment is most likely to be successful when the motivation for treatment comes from the patient rather than being imposed on the patient.

In 2023, the Canadian Society of Addiction Medicine reviewed studies on the effectiveness of compulsory treatment. Of twenty-two studies that compared compulsory to voluntary treatment, ten found negative outcomes from involuntary treatments, while just seven of them found better outcomes consisting of a greater likelihood of staying in treatment.

Consultant psychiatrists have told Pirzada that involuntary treatment for opioid use disorder isn't an option. "It's just a very sad situation," he told me. "It's something I wish we could see less of."

My own experience with Suboxone has been that it's effective but requires some investment of time over and above the initial patient assessment. You must try to shift patients like Theo-Joseph from reluctant to willing to take the medication, and once that shift has been made, you still have to coach them on how to take it.

Patient consults in the ER these days are dominated by cruel arithmetic. Decades ago, when I started practice, ER physicians would typically see anywhere from two to five patients each hour. In 2023, according to a US survey published in the *Western Journal of Emergency Medicine*, the median working pace was just 2.1 patients per hour.

My workflow would be much more efficient if I could see patients just once before sending them on their way. Prescribing Suboxone almost always means a fairly lengthy second session with the patient. I'm not against the extra time spent, but it's a reminder that every additional minute spent with one patient is a minute less for all the others.

Without comprehensive drug rehabilitation programs, administering and prescribing Suboxone may at times be an exercise in futility because it's about harm reduction and little else. Dr. Vincent Lam might agree with that. When I wrote *The Night Shift* in 2010, Lam was an ER colleague (and fellow author) in Toronto. In the years since, Lam departed the ER and became an addiction-medicine physician and the medical director of the Coderix Medical Clinic, an addictions clinic that focuses on helping people with difficulties around opioid use.

In 2024, Lam wrote an opinion piece for *The Globe and Mail* in which he argued that while harm reduction is essential to saving lives and reducing the suffering of patients, it is not a sufficient aim for people with opioid use dependency. He wrote, "It is crucial that harm-reduction programs, which aim to reduce illness, suffering and death while people are using drugs, channel people toward treatment and recovery."

The problem with that prescription is that there is a chronic lack of treatment programs in many parts of Canada.

Still, Lam reminds us that he was and still is a colleague to ER physicians. "When I was an emergency doctor, I performed cardiac resuscitations on people who'd suffered heart attacks so they would survive to receive treatment to open blockages in their hearts. A patient who needs multiple cardiac resuscitations and does not receive definitive treatment will soon die. Similarly, while overdoses need to be reversed, that effort will only have lasting impact if it leads people toward treatment."

Recently, the danger from fentanyl has taken a new and deadly turn. In April 2023, the US Office of National Drug Control Policy identified a veterinary tranquilizer called xylazine as an "emerging threat" when mixed with fentanyl. It was the first time the office had used that designation, which opens up a suite of measures designed to stop the spread of the drug, since it was created in 2019.

Xylazine was approved for veterinary use in 1971. It cannot be purchased without a veterinary licence. It goes by the trade names Rompun and Anased, but some of its street names are tranq and tranq dope. It has also been called the "zombie drug" because the combination of xylazine and fentanyl renders people unable to move, with no recall of what happened.

According to a drug alert put out by the Canadian Centre on Substance Use and Addiction and the Canadian Community Epidemiology Network on Drug Use, xylazine was first identified in the unregulated drug supply in Canada in 2012. It has been found in samples of fentanyl, cocaine and methamphetamine. People reportedly use it to prolong the effects of these drugs. Xylazine is extremely dangerous because it can lower the heart rate, blood pressure and breathing rate. Combining it with opioids and other central nervous system depressants like benzodiazepines or alcohol can significantly slow these vital functions, increasing the risk of overdose and death. Injecting xylazine is also associated with "tranq wounds," which are severe skin ulcers that sometimes necessitate amputations.

And here's the kicker: Naloxone has no effect on xylazine. In fact, there is no known antidote to the drug.

Dr. Carolyn Snider has seen the new danger up close. The ER physician at St. Michael's Hospital who we met earlier in the book says St. Mike's is ground zero of the new and more dangerous opioid crisis.

"It just happens all day, every day," Snider said. "It's not uncommon to have four or five overdoses in an eight-hour shift." She told me that even as we were talking, she had two patients in the ER who needed to be resuscitated at the same time. "Two guys found down at the same time shared the same dealer and they both had prolonged low heartbeats," she said. The slow heart rate and low blood pressure these patients have is so profound that even once they're resuscitated, they need to be watched closely. "If they have bradycardia"—abnormally low heart rate—"we probably need to keep them on our monitors." Also, the sleepiness often lasts many hours after the heart and breathing rates and blood pressure return to normal. "Once they're breathing regularly, they could be off a monitor for a while," she explained. "But it's going to take them eighteen hours of sleep to wake up . . . They will likely be on our monitors for many hours today. I'm going to guess probably into the late evening."

It's important to remember that not everyone who uses fentanyl plus contaminants like xylazine lives to tell about it.

According to the Centers for Disease Control, xylazine has been implicated in an increasing number of drug-related deaths in the US. In 2018, there were just 102 deaths involving xylazine, but by 2021, that number had skyrocketed to about 3,500. Over 99 per cent of the xylazine-related deaths also involve fentanyl.

Xylazine is starting to take hold in Canada. The federal Drug Analysis Service tests drug samples submitted by public health agencies and police. In 2024, 12.6 per cent of opioid samples contained xylazine—twice as much as in the year before.

The 2022 Community Epidemiology Network drug alert cited an uptick in reports of xylazine-laced fentanyl in BC, Manitoba, Ontario, Quebec and Nova Scotia. Some jurisdictions are examining samples at the local level. Toronto's Drug Checking Service found that xylazine was found in 55 per cent of the expected fentanyl samples tested in a two-week period in March 2025. That is by far the service's highest proportion of tranq-containing samples.

Ontario's Office of the Chief Coroner reported that there were few if any deaths connected to xylazine before 2020. From 2021 to 2023, xylazine was detected in 184 drug toxicity deaths. In 2024, there were many media reports about xylazine turning up in communities across Canada. For example, there were twenty-two suspected xylazine-related deaths in Ottawa in the first four weeks of the year. And in February, a cocktail of fentanyl, xylazine and a benzodiazepine was blamed for triggering nearly two dozen overdoses in Belleville, a small city just off the main highway between Toronto and Montreal. There were no deaths in that case, but the pressure put on first responders was so great that the city declared a state of emergency.

St. Mike's has become such an important player in the battle to save patients who use fentanyl that the hospital has opened a lab to act as Toronto's drug-checking service. People can go there to get timely and detailed information on what's in their drugs before they take them. The service is anonymous and non-stigmatizing, and it exists to help users make informed decisions. It also shares information on Toronto's unregulated drug supply with harm-reduction workers and clinicians to help them refine the care they provide and to facilitate research and policy development.

The addiction crisis is a saga without end. As soon as doctors, nurses, paramedics and harm-reduction workers start to get a handle on one new drug, another pops up to replace it. This is what happened in early 2024, when Toronto Public Health put out an alert about a disturbing threefold increase in suspicious opioid-related deaths in the last week of February. The deaths were believed to be related not to xylazine but to new tranquilizers called medetomidine and dexmedetomidine. These are non-opioid medications used as sedatives and pain relievers and are more potent than xylazine. Combined with fentanyl and xylazine, they slow breathing and lower blood pressure and heart rate.

Around the same time, Toronto Public Health also reported detecting high concentrations of fluorofentanyl in the city's street supply. Fluorofentanyl has the same effect on the body as fentanyl but is up to five times more potent. That increases the risk of accidental overdose for users. For rescuers, it means even larger doses of naloxone may be required to save individuals experiencing an overdose.

5:30 a.m.

"Brian, go to resus stat!" Vivica's voice on the intercom sounds edgy. I take off for the resuscitation room, frantically wondering which patient of mine has gone south in a hurry.

The first thing that greets me as I enter the room is the unmistakable odour of dead and infected tissue. Putrid and vaguely sweet-smelling at the same time.

I instinctively switch to mouth breathing as I scramble to don a fresh N95 mask, gown, gloves and face shield. Thankfully, the mask quickly blocks the smell. As I walk into the resuscitation room, Samir, the night doctor, is treating Circe. She's the woman I briefly met as the paramedics wheeled her into the ER with a possible bacterial infection in her bloodstream. Woody, a veteran respiratory therapist, is prepping BiPAP (short for bilevel positive airway pressure), an airway and breathing device that pushes pressurized air into the lungs via a mask connected to a ventilator. BiPAP helps patients breathe in more oxygen and breathe out more carbon dioxide when the effort is tiring them out.

Rishna and Lance, the resuscitation nurses, work fast to prime two IV infusion devices.

"How much norepinephrine do you want?" Lance asks Samir.

"Start at ten micrograms per minute," he replies. "Check BP every two minutes.

"Samir," I say as I walk into the room, "I figure Circe is septic, but what's the source?"

"She is ten days post-surgery," says Samir. "She got silicone breast implants in Brazil. She got back five days ago and had a low-grade fever for three days plus chills and chest pain. Her roommate called 911. Her chest is bruised, and the breast implant incisions are partially open and oozing pus."

That explains the odour I detected. It's coming from pus and dead tissue surrounding the implants. Samir is painting an ominous picture. Fever, chills, chest pain and bruising plus discharge can mean only one thing: The breast implants have become infected. Worse than that, she may be developing sepsis.

"Have you been taking antibiotics?" I ask Circe. Post-implant infections occur when the surgical wound is contaminated with bacteria or fungi. Most infections like this take hold up to a week following surgery.

"They gave me a prescription which I filled at the clinic in Brasilia." Her voice is muffled by the breathing mask she wears and the hiss of oxygen coming from a wall unit. "I finished the last one three days ago."

"You've started IV antibiotics?" I ask Samir.

"Already given," he replies. "I also ordered two litres of IV fluid. As soon as I gave it, Circe's blood pressure started trending down. When she arrived, her BP was 105 over 70. Now, it's 88 over 65. Her oxygen saturation is also down. It was 98 per cent when she arrived. Now, it's 92 per cent."

This is where medicine gets complicated. We know that sepsis causes the blood pressure to crash. The toxins produced by the infection make the blood vessels dilate and become leaky. That causes the fluid inside the blood vessels to leak into the surrounding tissues, lowering the blood pressure. To compensate for that, we were taught to give patients many litres of intravenous fluid. If a patient's blood pressure dropped after getting IV fluids, we thought it meant that she needed more fluids.

But more recently, we've learned that is not necessarily the case. Often, too much fluid does more harm than good. That's because sepsis also causes the heart muscle to fail. If the heart muscle stops pumping forcefully, the fluids back up into the lungs, causing congestion and respiratory distress.

"Does Circe need more fluid or less?" I'm asking myself as much as anyone else in the room.

"Could you whip out your ultrasound probe and check the heart?" says Samir.

"Circe, I'm going to do a quick ultrasound of your heart," I tell her. "Is that okay?"

She nods.

Circe winces as I squirt an inch of gel onto her chest and then cries out when I gently place the probe on the bruised area. Samir and I exchange a knowing glance. Doctors call that exaggerated reaction to a mildly uncomfortable test "pain out of proportion." When pressing on a patient causes far more pain and distress than might be expected, it can indicate necrotizing fasciitis, or flesh-eating disease. The worst possible infection imaginable.

"I'll try to make this as quick as I can," I tell her as I inch the probe on the left side of her chest, as wide of the left implant as I can go while still getting an image. "Just a few more seconds."

Samir and I both look at the image of Circe's heart on my phone. If her left ventricle collapses with each heartbeat, it means she needs lots more fluids. But that's not what her echo shows.

"The left ventricle appears dilated," I tell Samir. "The muscle is hardly moving with each beat."

"Circe, the echo shows that the infection is affecting your heart," Samir tells her. "I'm going to start a medication to get your heart muscle to work better."

"How much dobutamine do you want me to start?" Lance asks. Dobutamine stimulates receptors that make heart muscle cells contract more forcefully. It is given by IV drip.

"Let's start at eighty micrograms per minute," says Samir. "That's one microgram per kilogram per minute."

"Rishna, can you give Circe a milligram of IV hydromorphone?" Samir orders.

"Are you concerned about her blood pressure?"

Rishna is right to question Samir's order. IV opioids like hydromorphone can drop a patient's blood pressure. Not a great outcome at this moment.

"I am," Samir replies, "but I'd rather treat her pain and watch her BP carefully than let her suffer." He turns his attention back to Circe. "I'm pretty sure you have a serious infection involving your breast implants," he tells her. "I'm calling the general surgeons to come and see you. Because the infection involves your chest, I'm also calling the chest surgeons. And I'm admitting you to the ICU, where they can keep a close watch on you."

"I went all the way to Brazil for this," says Circe, in pain and in tears.

Circe had her breast implants in Brazil. It's up to healthcare workers in Canada to manage the complications.

This is not an isolated situation. According to the 2022 annual global survey on aesthetic/cosmetic procedures by the International Society of Aesthetic Plastic Surgery, Brazil performs more cosmetic surgical procedures than any other country in the world.

Many of those who get those procedures are "medical tourists," people who travel outside their own country to receive medical procedures and other kinds of healthcare at cheaper costs than they could get in Canada. A subset of these patients are called "cosmetic tourists" because they seek cosmetic surgical procedures.

According to statista.com, in 2023, 1.8 per cent of Canadian patients received treatment outside of the country. Gynecological and orthopedic procedures were among the most sought treatments by Canadians going abroad.

In 2022, the top five surgical cosmetic procedures were liposuction, breast augmentation, eyelid surgery, abdominoplasty and breast lift. The most popular non-surgical procedures were Botox injections, hyaluronic acid injections, hair removal, chemical peel and non-surgical fat reduction. Botox is the most common non-surgical procedure for both men and women and across all age groups.

Those statistics are increasingly meaningful to physicians like

Dr. Ian Chernoff. He is one of the most respected ER physicians in Toronto, with broad experience in academic and community emergency medicine. He also happens to be an expert in point-of-care ultrasound. If Samir and I know how to scan Circe's heart, it's because Ian Chernoff taught us. He is certified as a master instructor by the Canadian Point of Care Ultrasound Society, the premier organization in Canada for training physicians in bedside ultrasound.

Recently, Chernoff has noticed that his shifts are dotted with patients who got cosmetic procedures outside the country and have turned to local ERs to manage the complications. "I've had several that come to mind," he told me. "A woman who had gone to a Central American country for liposuction and developed a very serious skin infection after the procedure, and came back to Canada and presented to the emergency department to try to receive care."

Unlike Circe, that patient did not have flesh-eating disease. "It wasn't quite as serious as that," said Chernoff. "But it was bad enough that [she] needed to be admitted to hospital for intravenous antibiotics."

Deciding that a patient needs to be admitted to receive antibiotics is the easy part. Finding a specialist who will admit the patient is a lot more challenging.

"It was a huge problem trying to figure out which service would take the patient," Chernoff recalled. "The surgical services were reluctant to do so because they hadn't performed the procedure."

In medicine, there is a kind of golden rule, something that is passed down from physician to physician: The surgeon who does the operation manages the complications. This means you take care of your patient when things go wrong, and if somebody else did the procedure, they should manage their own complications. It's part of being a good colleague.

Some of this is simply financial, even though it's not often talked about in a publicly funded healthcare system. The cosmetic surgeon gets paid a lot of money to do the original surgery, and there is an argument to be made that the fee the patient paid should include managing any complications. The surgeon on call to the ER physician works in the publicly funded system and is therefore paid far less to fix whatever's gone wrong. Obviously, Circe's surgeon in Brazil would not be available to manage her unfortunate complication.

Another issue has to do with the patients and their new reality. They go from choosing the procedure and the cosmetic surgeon to having little or no choice at all. They go from expecting to look better to hoping at best to salvage what was done and at worst to avoid looking like they've come from a war zone. It takes a special surgeon to guide a patient through all that.

Chernoff also pointed out that surgeons like to do operations, but in the case of his patient, "there wasn't another surgical procedure to be done." He says the surgeon he approached asked him to refer the patient to another kind of specialist instead. "They asked me to speak to the internal medicine service to admit the patient to hospital, which ultimately they did," Chernoff explained. "But dealing with post-operative infections is not their expertise. They shouldn't be tasked with dealing with these sorts of things."

That Chernoff's patient was a cosmetic tourist presented yet another challenge. "The woman who came back from Central America had no documentation of the sort of procedure that had been done," he said. "It really hampered the ability to provide care for her."

Then there's the fact that the patient has probably spent a lot of money going abroad for cosmetic surgery. A survey of Canadians who went to other countries for cosmetic procedures published in 2022 in the journal *Plastic Surgery* found that the average outlay was $11,495. Most paid travel costs on top of that. That's still cheaper than the domestic cost.

The more people spend, the greater their expectations that things will turn out okay no matter the complications. Imagine being the ER physician who has to explain to Circe that those costly breast implants need to be removed less than a week after being put in.

"There's a huge mismatch there," said Chernoff. "What their goals of care are might be quite different than mine. They've spent a lot of money to travel somewhere to have a procedure done. They want that procedure salvaged by any means possible. My goal is for them to be well and to get better. There are some situations where we might have to make an incision into a cosmetic surgical procedure that's been done in a very fancy way by a plastic surgeon abroad."

It's one thing to have to manage the complications from procedures done abroad. It's quite another to take care of a patient whose procedure was done across town. But that's exactly what Chernoff is also observing in the ER.

"I saw a woman with a filler she'd had injected into her face," he said. "She told me it was done at an aesthetic clinic by a nurse, under the delegation of a family physician." The patient had a facial infection. "The filler was in fact oozing out of the pores in her cheek. It looked rather like caulking around your sink." He asked the patient what she was told to do in the event of complications. He found the answer disturbing. "She was lost," he told me. "She had contacted the clinic for next steps, but there was nothing offered to her at all."

Chernoff suspects that the medical director at the clinic lacked the surgical training needed to deal with the infection that arose. And when the patient wasn't given any help, she didn't know what else to do but go to the emergency department. Once again, he found himself stuck in the position of having to try to persuade a specialist to come to the aid of the patient. "I spoke to the plastic surgeon on call," he said. "They weren't really interested in seeing the patient in the emergency department. They said I could send off a referral to the plastic surgery outpatient clinic. And I did that. But I don't really know what the outcome was."

Sometimes, the complications that bring patients to the ER come from procedures done decades ago by esteemed local cosmetic surgeons who have long since retired. Chernoff cites another patient who had filler injected into her face, but in this case, the filler was later banned by Health Canada. "We did a CT scan that showed that she had a significant infection, and the filler had become enmeshed in the tissues of her face."

Chernoff asked several specialists to see the patient, starting with the plastic surgeon on call. All told him the problem wasn't theirs to treat. After the fourth call—and feeling increasingly desperate—he decided to try the on-call plastic surgeon a second time. "And on my second call, they agreed to come and see the patient."

A big part of our jobs as ER physicians is persuading specialists to come and see our patients. We tend to get better at it with age and experience, but it's always time-consuming. There is nothing more frustrating to us than having to repeat the same request to three or four different specialists and to be told no each time.

These kinds of interactions lead to stress among ER physicians. They also lead to moral injury, or a sense that your moral or ethical code has been violated. But what bothers us the most is the measurable risk that the patient with complications is harmed by delayed care and the lack of definitive care. Ian Chernoff has yet another case with a bearing on that.

The patient had several cosmetic surgery procedures done at a private plastic surgery hospital in Toronto. But one, a procedure called a tracheal shave—sometimes referred to as "Adam's apple surgery"—went wrong. Adam's apple surgery is often requested by trans women and non-binary people who want a more feminine appearance. It may also be done on cisgender women who want the same effect.

In rare circumstances, the procedure can injure the trachea, and that's what happened to Chernoff's patient. "At the end of the procedure, the surgeon noticed that the patient had extensive subcutaneous emphysema," he told me. Subcutaneous emphysema means that air is getting into tissues directly underneath the skin. The affected skin often appears swollen and is tender to the touch. When you press on it, the air under the skin has a crinkly feeling and sounds like bubble wrap. The most common locations for subcutaneous emphysema are in the skin covering the neck or chest, though it can also occur in other parts of the body.

In this case, the surgeon was concerned that the tracheal shave had injured the windpipe, causing air to leak into the neck. Such injuries are relatively benign in most cases, but they can lead to life-threatening complications, including collapsed lungs and mediastinitis, a condition in which the space containing the heart in the middle of the chest becomes inflamed or infected. "If the patient had a collapsed lung they could have the same findings under their skin," said Chernoff.

The clinic was closing for the day and the surgeon, concerned that the air leak would continue, sent the patient to the ER. "The lights are going off, and everyone's going home," Ian surmised. "So they really had nowhere to send the patient, and the patient was clearly not well enough to be discharged home. They really had no action plan as to what to do."

As an ER physician like me, Chernoff is not an expert in this kind of injury. Still, once the patient arrived in the ER, it became his duty to provide care. Fearing a life-threatening complication, he brought the patient to the resuscitation room and requested a CT scan of the neck and the chest. The CT showed that the surgeon was probably right. "In all likelihood the air leak was coming from the trachea," said Chernoff, "which is a less serious possibility and not one of the more dangerous life-threatening possibilities."

Chernoff asked the ear, nose and throat surgeon on call to see the patient and got no pushback. But there was a catch. "They didn't want to admit the patient to one of their beds," he recalled. "I do understand it from their perspective. It's a procedure they don't do. And if they admit the patient to one of their beds, they have to cancel one of their elective surgeries the next morning. Whatever the reasons, the ENT surgeon was kind enough to tell me that there wasn't a life-threatening problem. And then the patient was left to us in the emergency department to manage overnight."

And that's what they did. "We pride ourselves as emergency providers on being able to manage a broad range of medical problems," he said. "But this patient probably should have been admitted to a surgical stepdown unit—maybe even a surgical ICU."

The patient remained stable overnight. The next morning, after the plastic surgery clinic reopened, Chernoff transferred the patient back there in an ambulance. As far as he knows, the problem resolved on its own, and no further treatment was required.

One of the reasons why Chernoff was keen to talk to me was to offer a warning to the growing ranks of people who are having cosmetic procedures.

"I have no doubt that many times things go swimmingly and there [are] no problems," he told me. "I just worry that people really don't know what they're getting into if things go wrong. If you go to a clinic with a full range of services and a cosmetic surgeon who can address complications, that's one thing. But if you've gone with perhaps a more economical approach, and there's no one within the clinic that can fix it, I think patients may be spending a whole lot more money than they're bargaining for. And it's going to be something that they're going to have to navigate on their own."

The ER is the one place in the system that can't say no to any patient. But Dr. Ian Chernoff wonders if managing the rare and exotic complications of cosmetic surgery is a task too far.

CHAPTER TWELVE

DESPAIR

5:45 a.m.

Ahu comes towards the triage station. Her usually open and expressive face is blank, her hands clenched into fists.

"Tired?" I ask her.

"I'm fine," she replies in an unconvincing way.

"Sometimes the guy at Starbucks starts early," I tell her. "Coffee on me?"

Ahu doesn't make eye contact as we walk silently to the coffee stand in the lobby. I resist the temptation to prod my resident as we take our coffees to the doctors' office in the ER. She'll tell me what's going on when she's ready.

"I should have sent you home an hour ago," I tell her.

She squeezes a couple of teardrops from her eyes. "I'm going to file a complaint," she finally says.

"What happened?" I ask her.

"I went to reassess Theo and to ask him again if he wanted to give Suboxone a try. He started yelling at me. It's like he snapped. He said I was judging him. He started calling me names. He used the N-word."

"I'm sorry."

"I'm used to it," she says, looking away. "Most of the time, I'm good at ignoring it. Maybe I'm tired."

"Do you want me to talk to him?"

She smiles at me. "You can't fight my battles for me."

"No, I can't. If it makes you feel any better, I've had lots of patients who take one look at me and decide I'm not to their liking. I remember one time when a colleague overheard a heated exchange between me and a patient. I walked away. A few minutes later, I saw that the colleague had taken over. The two of them were connecting. I felt useless. I felt shame."

"But you don't know what it feels like to be a physician who is female and Black."

"No, I don't."

Ahu stiffens her posture. "I need a few minutes to centre myself," she says. "Then I'll try to talk to him about what he said and how it affected me."

"I'm here if you want me to stand beside you."

"I appreciate that," she says.

Ahu's shoulders slump as she walks away. I don't know what lasting impact this episode will have on her. I don't know how much my words helped her, if at all.

The thing is, from medical school through residency and beyond, the message we get repeatedly is that we're not supposed to have limits. Today, more and more patients put that message to the test.

One colleague who has thought a lot about that is Dr. Catherine Varner. A decade or so into her career as an ER physician in downtown Toronto, she's learned how to tolerate being on the receiving end of verbal abuse from patients. "Sometimes, they just let it rip," she told me, and it is hostile and vicious. I usually let them go on for a bit—as long as it's not physically aggressive towards me—and then I try to find a place of common ground." But she acknowledged that she needed "seasoning" as a human being to be able to make that shift. "I think it's impossible for someone who is a year or two into their career," she said.

For Varner, becoming a parent helped. She said that staying up all night with a screaming toddler made her realize the screaming is more about the child's distress than the parent's inadequacies. I can relate to this. As I near retirement, I'm much better at listening, without reacting, to the angry outbursts of patients and their loved ones. When you work in an ER, staying calm in the face of anger is a necessary skill.

It wasn't always that way for me. In the early days of my career, I found it hard to empathize with the aging spouses and middle-aged children who came to the ER alongside loved ones with dementia and other frailties. But becoming a caregiver to my own parents and my sister (who had young-onset dementia) enabled me to see things from their point of view. Frankly, I'm surprised these days at how much frustration patients and their caregivers tolerate in the ER without yelling.

This is a view Varner seems to share. She thinks the system has a considerable track record of letting down patients, especially those with the greatest needs. "We used to have a functioning shelter system," she said. "We used to have a functioning home care system and a palliative care system that kept people out of hospital. We have watched the disintegration of some of those social webs and networks that kept people out of hospital."

In some cases, those social webs have disintegrated. In others, they weren't developed in the first place. That's what happened in the aftermath of what's been called the deinstitutionalization movement. Beginning in Canada in the 1960s, facilities that housed people with severe chronic mental illnesses were closed, and patients were discharged into the care of their families or to other kinds of residences based in the community, such as halfway houses and group homes. These closures were supposed to take place in tandem with the development of robust community mental health services, but those resources mostly failed to materialize.

Many social scientists have documented the ramifications of this movement. Some have looked at the direct impact of deinstitutionalization on ERs in Canada. For example, a paper on psychiatric emergency nurses in Winnipeg, published in 2005 in the *Journal of Emergency Nursing*, showed that mental health complaints made up as many as 15 per cent of all ER visits. And those patients tend to be repeat visitors. It's not uncommon to see people who present with both mental health and substance use issues. In a 2023 report, the CIHI said that of Canadians who visit the ER for help dealing with substance use and mental health problems, one in ten make four or more trips each year.

Dr. Carolyn Snider, the ER physician at St Michael's Hospital, has had a long-standing interest in patients who come to the emergency room with mental health issues. In particular, she's a big proponent of trying verbal and other techniques to de-escalate conflicts, even when a patient is acting violently. In the past, that's a situation that would have called for security staff and possibly the police. Frequently it would have meant ER physicians like me using straps to restrain patients and strong sedatives to put them to sleep.

"We've all got some non-violent communication training," Snider told me. That might mean, for example, acknowledging a patient's right to be frustrated with having to wait to see a psychiatrist or a social worker. It might mean acknowledging physical needs like hunger. "They haven't eaten in two days. Let's get them a bite to eat." Often, that approach works. But in chaotic ERs post-Covid, patients and sometimes even caregivers can easily be triggered to escalate their agitated or aggressive behaviour.

To make matters worse, many patients with serious chronic mental health problems are either homeless or live in precarious housing. You don't need to be a health planner to appreciate the impact that dissolving the social safety net has had on those people.

Dr. Andrew Boozary is a family doctor and the executive director of the University Health Network's social medicine program, an initiative to improve the quality of care for people who live in disadvantaged circumstances by partnering with community organizations to address issues such as poverty, social isolation, food insecurity and the lack of affordable housing. Boozary has gathered statistics that connect the dots between frequent visits to the ER and lack of fundamental social supports. In a 2024 article in *Toronto Life,* he said that in 2019–20, 234 patients visited UHN's ER more than 15,000 times. That is an astonishing figure that works out to each patient visiting more than once a week, every week of the year. Boozary told the magazine that most of those "super users" were homeless.

"Many of my unhoused patients with diabetes struggle to manage their condition," he told *Toronto Life*. "Without stable housing, it's nearly impossible for them to store or consistently take insulin, leading to severe complications. On numerous occasions, I've even seen patients lose limbs to amputation."

That's bad for patients, bad for ERs and bad for the entire healthcare system. Boozary says lack of stable housing means the cost of healthcare for those patients goes up sevenfold.

Not content to talk challenges, Boozary is creating solutions. In 2024, UHN, in partnership with all three levels of government, opened Dunn House, a modular housing complex that's been described as Canada's first social medicine housing project. Dunn House is Boozary's baby. Now fully occupied, the complex provides stable, permanent and affordable housing—plus healthcare—to 51 of those 234 people who are the most frequent users of UHN's emergency departments, at about a tenth of the cost of a hospital visit. As reported in the *Toronto Star*, a $2-million expansion of the program will see services provided for up to another 100 people leaving homelessness. Boozary says the residents are chosen based on how often they've used the ER, how often and for how long they were admitted to hospital and other factors. "We reached out to individuals and extended invitations rather than taking applications," he told *Toronto Life*.

Dunn House isn't just a place to call home. The facility is also meant to address the full gamut of social and healthcare needs. Each resident has a studio apartment with a bathroom and a kitchen. There's also a community kitchen for making communal meals, plus common areas for social programs and a garden. Healthcare providers such as family doctors, nurse practitioners, social workers and psychiatrists are available on-site.

This is not a completely new idea. An article on healthydebate.ca, a site focused on healthcare journalism, looked at programs in other countries that involved providing accommodations to patients whose housing is precarious. The authors cited a Chicago study that identified clients with no fixed address who, when discharged from hospital, were given a secure roof over their head provided by the city. The results were an impressive 24 per cent drop in ER visits and a nearly 30 per cent reduction in days spent in hospital.

Since Dunn House has just recently welcomed its first tenants, it's way too soon to predict how successful the project will be in the long run. I love the big idea behind it, but I have my doubts about its long-term success. Critics will be watching and waiting to pounce should the complex become a hot spot for fentanyl and other drug trafficking and related criminal activity. But even if Boozary and his colleagues manage to avoid obvious pitfalls like that, the political headwinds against scaling and spreading the concept to other jurisdictions will be enormous.

Still, I wish the facility and the people behind it every success.

Dunn House is focused on the all-important issue of how to divert one hospital's super users, but that still leaves the everyday patients with serious mental health conditions (including substance use) and other issues that make them more prone to violence. Dr. Catherine Varner believes in de-escalation but draws the line at physical abuse. Unfortunately, violence directed at frontline healthcare providers in the ER is becoming much more common.

In an article published in 2022 in *CMAJ*, Samantha Marchand, an ER nurse at St. Mike's, reported that she and her colleagues have had patients toss "vomit, stool, urine, semen" onto them. She said that they have become numb to incidents of physical and verbal abuse, which happen on every shift. "It's something that's been normalized, and we are desensitized," she told the article's authors. What's more, she said the violence appeared to be increasing in understaffed and overwhelmed ERs.

Marchand's on-the-job observations were confirmed in a position statement published by the Canadian Association of Emergency Physicians in August 2021. "The problem of workplace violence in the emergency department is grave," read the statement. "Healthcare providers have an estimated four-fold higher rate of workplace violence and fully half of such attacks occur in the ED." Not surprisingly, nurses bear the brunt of those attacks. CAEP cited studies showing that more than half of ER nurses are physically or verbally abused in any given week.

There are plenty of recent examples of violence as well. In January 2025, two healthcare workers were stabbed at the Halifax Infirmary. A few months later, a nurse was strangled into unconscious at Vancouver General Hospital. And this is happening everywhere, not just in overcrowded urban ERs. Tiggy Baker, the former ER nurse at the Perth and Smiths Falls District Hospital in Perth, Ontario, told me that she was often on the receiving end of verbal and physical abuse. "In the two weeks before I left [the ER], I had a steel garbage can thrown onto the back of my head," she recalled. "I've been headbutted in the face. Dr. Al Drummond"—her colleague and the former ER chief—"was bitten on the arm by a patient as we were trying to put him into physical restraints. And it's not just the physical abuse. It's the verbal abuse."

Like many other ERs, the one in Perth put up signs saying that violence and verbal abuse would not be tolerated, but that was an ineffective deterrent. "The signs are a nice smokescreen," Tiggy said. "Realistically, at the end of the day, the patients don't care, and the police are overburdened."

Over my four decades and counting as an ER physician, I've heard and witnessed many incidents of patients verbally or physically assaulting ER nurses and other staff. In my experience, assaults against physicians are far less common, but that's changing.

In 2022, my colleague Dr. Qassim Tejpar was on the receiving end of an act of violence committed by a patient. It happened on a night shift.

"I was the only physician in the department," he explained to me. "I went to assess a patient who had come in by ambulance. He was lying in the stretcher in our waiting room. He had been brought in because he didn't want to get off of a transit vehicle, and he complained of some chest pain. And so the paramedics had brought him into the hospital."

Tejpar wasn't prepared for what happened next. "He looked pretty calm, and he was quiet when I approached him. I said hello, and he jumped out of his bed and punched me in the mouth." This occurred during the Covid pandemic, so Tejpar was wearing an N95 mask and a face shield. But even with all of that PPE, he still felt the impact. "I was tasting a little bit of blood in my mouth. And when I checked myself out later, I had a cut on my lip."

After the patient was detained and placed under the control of the hospital security team, Tejpar called the police. They arrived soon after and charged the patient with assault but released him into the care of the hospital security team. Tejpar experienced days of dental and facial pain. "I definitely had a concussion," he said. "For at least five or six days afterwards, I was experiencing headaches. I was extremely tired. I was having some trouble concentrating." He ended up missing four or five shifts of work.

Most ER physicians in Canada are self-employed, so that time off meant no income for Tejpar. There were also costs borne by his colleagues, who had to fill his missed ER shifts.

And there was another issue. Having just been assaulted, Tejpar felt he could not provide the patient with proper care. At the same time, however, he was wondering if the man's behaviour was caused by a medical condition that required treatment. "You've got a patient who's just assaulted you and yet you're still responsible for their medical care," he said. "You can't be impartial at that point. I knew that I couldn't provide him any sort of care after he hit me like that." With Tejpar the only physician on shift, there were no colleagues to see the patient instead of him. After several conversations with local law enforcement, they returned and took the patient to another ER to be assessed.

Tejpar's experience was shocking, but he's reluctant to call himself a victim, especially when he considers just how much more often ER nurses face verbal, physical and psychological abuse. "Nurses are huge victims of violence in the emergency department," he said. "My nursing colleagues suffer a lot. We've been hearing more and more from nurses over the past while, as things get harder for them, that something needs to change."

Tejpar has thought a great deal about why such incidents are on the rise. "I can say that we've definitely been seeing a trend towards more agitated people in our emergency departments," he told me. "People who lack patience, people who lack politeness or courtesy, people who are more willing to get into arguments and get into disagreements and people who are more demanding. I think there's a bit of an agitated state in the population. There seems to be a bit more permission to take it out on healthcare professionals. And I don't really know where that's come from."

I asked Tejpar if he thought the attack on him was racially motivated, but he said he had no way of knowing. I sensed that it was easier for him to talk about racism directed at colleagues. "I've definitely witnessed racially motivated violence in our department," he said. "Especially towards some of the nurses. It's horrible."

It's also an issue he thinks is not getting enough attention. "Nurses from minority groups experience verbal abuse more frequently," he noted. "Every week, I see incidents that are racially motivated. Insults and attacks on nurses who are just . . . doing their jobs. And it's really hard to watch."

I first spoke with Tejpar shortly after he was attacked. At that time, he was dealing with both the lingering concussion symptoms and the ongoing emotional fallout. He told me he was experiencing a sense of fear in situations that were similar to the one in which he was assaulted. During one shift, he got into an argument with a patient after performing a physical. "She didn't appreciate the diagnosis I gave her, and she got quite upset about it," he said. Despite the pushback, he stuck with his clinical opinion.

The patient then went to another physician, who agreed with her self-diagnosis. After that, she tracked down Tejpar on the phone and proceeded to tell him what she thought of his assessment skills. "She just started ripping me apart," he said. "I ended up having a panic attack on the phone. I had palpitations. I was having a hard time composing words. I had to stop talking, and it took about five minutes for it to get better."

That was the worst episode, but Tejpar told me there have

been others. He said he found it "exhausting" to deal with patients with severe complex mental health problems, and he also noticed changes in his demeanour off the job. "I think there was also spillover at home—getting upset more easily, feeling tired, those kinds of things." He now understands that he was suffering from burnout.

Studies have shown high rates of burnout—defined as feelings of energy depletion or exhaustion, increased mental distance from or feelings of negativism to one's job, and reduced professional efficacy—among ER physicians. It's tempting to believe that these claims are largely anecdotal, but when it comes to ER physicians in Canada, there's data to back them up.

A longitudinal survey of hundreds of ER doctors was carried out by the Network of Canadian Emergency Researchers, a not-for-profit group of mainly emergency room physicians whose goal is to conduct research to improve emergency patient care for all Canadians. The study was launched in April 2020, just as the pandemic was getting underway. Participants were invited to complete a weekly survey for ten weeks, with follow-up surveys that fall and two years later. The median age of participants was forty-two—meaning these were not physicians close to retirement but primarily those in the prime of their careers—and they were almost evenly split between men and women. Half of those who took part had been practising emergency medicine for twelve years or less.

Three hundred and nine participants completed surveys in 2020 and 2022, allowing for a valid comparison of burnout rates over the first two years of the pandemic. In 2022, scores for both emotional exhaustion and depersonalization (mental distance) went up significantly.

When asked if there was anything else they wanted to tell researchers about their experiences during the pandemic, participants listed things like disappointment in the system, lack of resources, lack of staff, working in a "horrible" environment, minimal hospital support and lack of government acknowledgment of the crisis. "The number of abusive patients is increasing all the time," wrote one respondent. "It is unfathomable that it is the front-line workers who have been showing up for our population throughout the pandemic that get the brunt of people's frustration with our broken health care system. Everyone deserves better. Patients and nurses and doctors, we all deserve better."

The survey results were published in 2024 in the *Annals of Emergency Medicine*, a top-ranked peer-reviewed journal for ER physicians. The authors' conclusion is sobering: "Our findings are a clear call for immediate government action to address the collapse of the emergency care system and for organizations to redress the negative impact experienced by emergency physicians when institutional support is lacking."

This survey was an eye-opener, but if anything, the rates of burnout among ER nurses are even worse. Dr. Catherine Varner says many of her nurse colleagues express the same frustrations and sense of despair. "A lot of those people have already left, to be quite frank," she told me. "Those of us who remain have come to terms with the fact that the next twenty years are going to be very difficult."

As weapons become more commonplace in violent attacks against ER and other healthcare providers, hospitals in Canada are taking preventive measures. Taking a page from the US, some hospitals here have installed metal detectors at ER and other entrances. Other hospitals have gone a step further, contracting with third-party providers to install weapons detection systems. These sophisticated systems combine advanced sensors and video systems with artificial intelligence to identify knives or guns and distinguish them from common pocketed items such as car and house keys.

In 2023, Windsor Regional Hospital became the first in Canada to install such a system. In the first year and a half after implementation, the hospital went from detecting ten weapons a year to finding thousands, including knives, brass knuckles and drug paraphernalia. Visitors seem to have gotten the message. The hospital has begun to see an overall drop in weapons found on visitors.

Other hospitals in Canada are taking note. After a shooting that took place in the ER at Victoria Hospital, London Health Sciences Centre, which operates the city's hospital network, became one of the latest to purchase a weapons detection system.

These days, Dr. Qassim Tejpar is feeling better about emergency medicine—and about himself. He reached that place in part by cutting back on ER shifts in downtown Toronto and spending more time working in smaller hospitals in rural and remote parts of Ontario. He said he needed "to get away from the environment in the city."

He says he's found solace outside the city. "I've been very happy doing it," he told me. "Rural medicine is really interesting. The patients are generally just happy that somebody's there. Their expectations are very different from a lot of patients in the city. The nurses seem a little less burnt-out."

6:00 a.m.

Ahu has a distraught look on her face. "He's gone," she says. "He left before I could talk with him. He pulled out his IV and left."

"A patient verbally assaults you and you're worried about the patient?" I ask her. "You're a smart MD with a good heart, Ahu, but you're also allowed to have boundaries."

"What if this was the time when he was ready to address his opioid use? And now the moment is gone."

"I doubt he was buying what you were selling. I've seen plenty of dope sickness, and I wouldn't wish it on my worst enemy. For Theo, entering recovery will be painful. Only he can decide when the pain of continuing his current path is greater than the pain of living without fentanyl and whatever else is mixed in with it."

I can't tell from Ahu's face whether she's about to cry or scream.

"You and I have both stayed much longer than the usual casino shift," I tell her. "Your work tonight was exceptional. I have a few patients to sort out, but you should go home and get some sleep."

"Okay," she says. "I want to check up on a couple of things, but then I promise to go."

As she turns away, I catch a look on her face. She's troubled that Theo left the ER without something positive coming from his visit. She's afraid something bad will happen to him, and it will be her fault. I know that look because I've felt it a thousand times.

CHAPTER THIRTEEN

HORIZON

6:10 a.m.

"You're actually sitting down," I say to Samir as I join him in the doctors' office. For most of the night, Samir and I have been in constant motion. But 6:00 a.m. means the colleague who is working the first shift of a new day is here, and that in turn means I don't have to see the next patient. I can exhale. Apparently, so can Samir.

He's looking at a CT scan of Circe's chest. She's the woman whose Brazilian breast implants have become infected.

"Thanks for staying," Samir replies without looking up from the screen. "Couldn't have made it through without you."

"Or Ahu," I remind him. I lean in to have a better look at the scan. "That doesn't seem good."

Samir points to some wavy white lines inside Circe's breast tissue. "Look at all that fat stranding."

Fat stranding is a term that radiologists invented to describe an area of fatty tissue that has streaks of white running through it. Those streaks are an ominous sign—they're what happens when the tiny vessels that carry lymphatic fluid become swollen and engorged. In this case, it means the breasts are chock-full of infection. Worse still, fat stranding on a CT scan is seen commonly in patients with necrotizing fasciitis, or flesh-eating disease.

"Yikes!" I say, briefly losing that equanimity that physicians are supposed to possess.

"There's more," he says, clicking several times on the keyboard to show me a view of the pectoral muscles located underneath Circe's left breast. He points to several small, irregular black semicircles.

"Hello, sleepyheads!" Fix bursts into the office carrying a cardboard tray loaded with several large cups of coffee. "I thought you might need a jolt."

"Fix, are you on days?" I grab one of the cups and add cream and a sweetener.

"I didn't figure on a short turnaround," he says, smiling as he looks at me in a teasing sort of way, "but someone made me stay late last evening. Wait." Fix's eyes widen as he looks at Circe's CT. "Are those gas bubbles in the chest wall?"

The lungs and the gastrointestinal tract are the only parts of the human body that are supposed to hold air bubbles. Gas does not belong deep inside the tissues of Circe's chest wall. It means her chest is infected with gas-producing bacteria. This, too, is a sign that she has necrotizing fasciitis caused by the infected breast implants.

The most powerful antibiotics known to doctors will not stop this galloping infection. The only chance to save Circe's life is for surgeons to rush her to the OR and remove as much as they can of the dead and dying infected tissue on her chest wall. And they have to do it as quickly as possible.

"How is Circe doing now?" I ask Samir.

"Her blood pressure is as stable as it's going to be," he says. "The surgeons and the anesthesiologist are prepping her for surgery."

"I'm going to start seeing patients," says Fix as he gets up to leave. "You two need to head home and get some sleep. Let me know when you're ready for handover."

Handover is what we do for any patient whose workup is not complete, who is waiting for test and X-ray results, by the time we go off shift. I tend to remain in the ER long after my shift has ended so that I can minimize the number of patients I need to hand over to someone else.

In more than four decades as an ER physician, I've participated in thousands of handovers. The one I'm about to tell you about, which took place in BC, is unlike any I have seen before.

It was 8:00 p.m., and Dr. Lindsey Dobson was finishing up a twelve-hour shift in the ER at Mackenzie and District Hospital and Health Centre, a five-stretcher ER in the small northern BC community of Mackenzie. But before Dobson could head home to grab some dinner and put her kids to bed, she had to hand over to Michael Ertel, the doctor on the night shift.

"I have four patients right now," said Dobson, who at that time had been a family physician in Mackenzie for more than a decade. "They're stable. I don't think you'll need to do very much with them. But I've decided to keep them in the ER overnight."

Four patients meant every stretcher but one in this tiny ER was full. The patients were typical of those you'd find in most ERs. The first was a young man who had been brought in by police with symptoms of psychosis, mainly agitation and the delusion that he could communicate with the devil.

"He tried to bite the nurse," Dobson told Ertel. Because of this, the man's arms and legs had been placed in restraints, but then he'd tried to use his body to strike one of the officers. Dobson said the man was so agitated he had to be sedated with a large dose of

nurses, but it's especially true for nurses in smaller and more rural hospitals, where they are often the only ones on duty. "After our medical clinic closes at 4 p.m. Monday to Friday," she told me, "our physicians are not on-site unless there's a reason that they're still here. We're pretty much solo most of the time after hours anyway, so that's not new to us at all." Pasichnyk and her fellow nurses have to be ready for anything. "We see all ages," she said. "We deal with obstetrical emergencies [and] psychiatric emergencies . . . there's a lot of motor vehicle accidents and things like that."

Ertel agrees that nurses are the linchpin. He told me one recent story about an older man who was experiencing dizziness and went to the Mackenzie ER because he thought he was having a stroke. Ertel suspected that the patient was actually suffering from an inner ear problem called benign paroxysmal positional vertigo, or BPPV. He had to make sure, though, because vertigo can also be a symptom of a stroke. And while BPPV is disturbing and nauseating, a stroke is life-threatening. Distinguishing between the two conditions is vitally important and requires a careful physical examination.

From his basement hundreds of kilometres away in Kelowna, Ertel asked the ER nurse to position the tablet so he could get a close look at the man's eyes. Then he told the nurse how to do a physical exam to elicit nystagmus, a type of involuntary eye movement seen with various causes of vertigo. Through that physical, Ertel was able to diagnose BPPV, which is the more benign condition and is caused by the presence of calcium particles in the fluid of the inner ear. The cure is to put the patient through a series of manipulations called the Epley manoeuvre to gradually move the particles to a part of the inner ear where they won't cause vertigo. With some coaching from Ertel, the nurse performed the procedure, and the patient got better. "It was pretty cool!" Ertel said. (If you're concerned that it's dangerous to have a doctor use a tablet to teach a nurse how to perform an Epley manoeuvre on a patient, I would point out that there are countless YouTube videos showing patients how to perform the manoeuvre on themselves.)

Ertel raves about the nurses he's worked with in the VERRa program. "None of these nurses signed up for this," he says. "They never thought they'd be working in a department where they're talking to a doctor on an iPad. But after two or three shifts, they say they're never going back to the pre-VERRa days."

British Columbia isn't the only province in Canada that's experimenting with virtual emergency medicine. Newfoundland and Labrador has also gone big on the idea. In 2023, the provincial government signed a two-year, $22-million deal with Teladoc Health Canada, a private company, to provide virtual care at select rural hospitals through its Virtual Emergency Room program. (Teladoc also provides virtual primary care for residents who don't have a family doctor.) The Dr. Y.K. Jeon Kittiwake Health Centre in New-Wes-Valley, a town on the east coast of Newfoundland, near Gander, was the first hospital in the province to sign up for the program. The hospital offers the virtual option when no physician is available to work in the ER. The program is similar to the one in BC, in that patients are first triaged and assessed by a nurse or advanced care paramedic and then seen virtually by an ER physician or nurse practitioner. But while the VERRa program hires physicians who live and practise in BC, Teladoc's VEC program uses doctors who are licensed to practise in Newfoundland and Labrador but may work and live in other provinces.

Dr. Cal Bergen is one of them. Bergen works as an ER physician at Victoria Hospital in Winnipeg but started doing virtual shifts for Teladoc in late 2023. On *White Coat, Black Art*, he said he works forty to fifty hours a month seeing patients virtually in Newfoundland and Labrador from his home office in Winnipeg. The interface between patient and virtual MD, Bergen explained, is a high-tech instrument that features a high-definition camera, a directional microphone and a speaker system, all operated by a touchscreen. A digital stethoscope and a digital otoscope (for examining the ear canal) allow Bergen to do a surprisingly detailed physical examination from many thousands of kilometres away. "I can listen to heart sounds and lung sounds," he explained. "I can look at the eardrums. I can look at throats and identify a strep throat. I can see these things and I can hear these things as clearly as I can when I'm in person at the Victoria Hospital." Bergen can also order blood tests and diagnostic imaging. His Newfoundland and Labrador medical licence permits him to prescribe medications. When necessary, he can transfer a patient from the rural hospital he's supporting to a larger hospital in a centre like Gander or St. John's.

Virtual emergency medicine even offers advantages that traditional in-person medicine cannot. When I'm on duty in my physical ER, I'm a blur of activity looking after ten or more patients, interacting with nurses, residents, nurse practitioners and physician assistants and fielding calls from specialists. Often, I have just five minutes to assess a patient before I get interrupted or distracted. The VERRa program, by contrast, doesn't run physicians like Dr. Ertel off their feet. On each shift, they serve only one remote ER. Ertel sees just one virtual patient at a time. (The physicians who work for Teladoc Health Canada may be seeing patients virtually at multiple sites.)

"I also think VERRa works really well for psychiatric patients," Ertel told me. "I have a lot more time to spend with the patient than I do in the emergency department when I've got twenty-five people waiting to see me. I feel pretty good about that."

Ertel was skeptical when he was approached about becoming one of VERRa's inaugural virtual ER doctors, but he's had so many positive encounters with patients that it's made him a convert. That includes a time when he managed virtually a young child with a peanut allergy whose parents brought him to a local ER. "I never thought I'd be talking on an iPad to parents and reassuring them that this is actually good care," he told me with a hint of awe.

In the months since Michael Ertel became a virtual ER physician, he's called the local family doctor back to the hospital on only one occasion. He takes seriously his role in giving an overworked family physician a night off. "We're dealing with underserviced areas that are hard to keep open," he told me. "There are too few family doctors who get to get home for a night's sleep every once in a while."

On the night in question, Dr. Ertel took over from a young family doctor. Just after the young doctor headed home, a fourteen-year-old girl with severe asthma was brought to the hospital by her parents. As part of his virtual assessment, Ertel checked the girl's electronic medical record, and that's how he learned that six months earlier, she'd had to be intubated and admitted to the ICU on a ventilator. That told Ertel that this young teen could develop severe respiratory distress in a hurry.

At this point, Ertel hadn't even seen the teen, but already he was worried. The nurse on duty brought a tablet to the patient's bedside. Ertel could see that the child was wheezing and breathing rapidly. He thought the child looked relatively well, but he noticed that her parents had fearful looks on their faces. He imagined the parents thinking, "I hope this guy's a good doctor. I hope he knows what he's doing. The nurses seem to know what they're doing, but my child's not getting better."

Ertel has thirty years of experience managing kids and adults with severe asthma, so he was confident in his ability to care for the girl. Relying on the nurse on scene to carry out his treatment plan, he ordered repeated doses of medications to relax her tight airways in order to help the girl breathe easier, as well as a corticosteroid to reduce the inflammation in her airways and lessen the amount of sticky mucus clogging them. Despite aggressive treatment, though, the girl's oxygen saturation started dropping, which meant she was still in respiratory distress. None of his interventions were breaking the asthma attack.

Dr. Ertel told me he started to feel anxious because he wasn't at the girl's bedside. On a typical virtual night shift, he would grab a bit of sleep between patients, but on this night, he was constantly on his tablet, checking the girl's vital signs. He was uneasy watching the scene unfold from hundreds of kilometres away and thought about summoning the family doctor he'd sent home but ruled it out. "It's always patient care first," said Ertel. "But there is that little bit of guilt in calling the doctor to come back. I think there's a little bit of pride. I'm the experienced doctor. Why do I need help?"

Around five in the morning, Ertel began to change his mind. He'd used every trick in the book to break the girl's asthma attack, to no avail. The nurse on scene had started to worry that the child was going to have a cardiac arrest. She asked Ertel several times if he wanted to call the local doctor back to the hospital. The fourth time she asked, it grabbed Ertel's attention. "My spidey senses are tingling here," he said. "I don't want to have to ask the local doctor on call to race to the hospital to do a crash intubation."

Ertel did decide to call the local doctor back to the hospital. The young physician arrived quickly, but ironically, he was less worried about the child than Ertel was. It turns out he had seen her during a previous asthma attack, when she looked in far worse distress. Instead of intubating her, the less experienced doctor kept watch by the bedside and continued to administer treatments to try to break the attack. It took a few more hours, but eventually the child's breathing eased, and she relaxed. She was admitted to the tiny hospital overnight and went home the next day without needing intubation or transport to a larger hospital.

Dr. Ertel's compelling anecdote is set against an increasingly spirited public debate on the viability and future of virtual emergency medicine. The whole notion of a not-quite-there ER is a topic of concern and criticism. Much of that criticism comes from emergency physicians themselves.

Dr. Michael Herman, an ER physician at Queensway Carleton Hospital in Ottawa, acknowledges that virtual care helps keep smaller ERs from closing. "I certainly have a lot of sympathy for these communities where you're really trying to plug a hole," he told me. "But I don't know if it's quite enough for what the communities need, to be honest."

Herman believes that most Canadians want to be seen in person by a physician who can look directly into their eyes and physically touch them to make a diagnosis. "Could you imagine talking to an iPad telling you that you had a cancer diagnosis?" Herman asked rhetorically. "You want to be sitting in the room with that person holding their hand, being a present physician."

In 2024, the Canadian Association of Emergency Physicians weighed in on the debate with a two-page position statement. The organization said there is a role for virtual care, particularly in consulting with and otherwise assisting doctors in remote ERs and facilities like primary care clinics. But CAEP also emphasized that "there are many instances in emergency care where in-person EP [emergency physician] assessment and interventions cannot be replaced by [virtual care]." The statement also made the critical point that the public expects an emergency department to have an ER physician available "to competently manage unexpected and time-sensitive illnesses or injuries. Unless an EP with competencies in emergency care is available to provide in-person assessment and treatment, the facility must not be labeled an ED."

Dr. Al Drummond, the venerable ER physician at the Perth and Smiths Falls District Hospital in Perth, Ontario, has been blunt in his denunciation of virtual emergency medicine. When Newfoundland and Labrador Health Services announced the virtual ER at Dr. Y.K. Jeon Kittiwake Health Centre in New-Wes-Valley, he posted on X about the "misinformation" on how healthcare works in Canada. According to Drummond, there simply "is no such FUCKING THING as a VIRTUAL ER!"

Ertel told me that while he shares Drummond's view that Canadian bricks-and-mortar ERs need more resources, he also sees a role for the virtual option, especially when it comes to a choice between virtual doctors and closing down a small ER. "I have a lot of respect for Al, and I take what he says very seriously, but I respectfully disagree with him on this," he said. He noted that Canada has never trained more physicians than it does now, and yet service has never been scarcer. "We've got to figure that out," he stressed. "Maybe it's time to think outside the box, and maybe it's time to look at other options."

Ertel has been on the front lines of virtual emergency medicine and has seen it succeed. "It's good care," he told me. "The patients, they love it. The nurses love it. The doctors love it. There's a lot of good people out there doing this, and they care just as much about the patients as [in-person doctors] do."

One physician who needs no convincing about the value of virtual medicine is Dr. Ray Markham. He's a family doctor in Valemount, a village of about eleven hundred people on the edge of the Rocky Mountains in northern BC. Markham does not work in an ER. Unlike Mackenzie, Valemount has no hospital. "The nearest CT scanner and emergency room would be three hundred kilometres away," Markham explained, "which is three hours' drive on a good day, and impossible to get to at times."

Originally from Zimbabwe, Markham first worked in Newfoundland and Labrador before moving to Valemount and opening a family practice in 2002. The lack of easy access to healthcare services in small and remote communities like his led him to become an early adopter of virtual medicine back then, except no one called it "virtual" at the time.

"We just started with radios," Markham recalled. "Then it was cellphones. Then we moved to video, probably ten or fifteen years ago. We've been doing experiments as to how we can make this work, be sustainable . . . I think there are many examples of rural people trying to make things work and not being comfortable with the status quo. It's really out of a necessity that comes from having to rely on each other and work together."

What drove these early experiments was not a need for big-city clinical expertise but a desire to pool scarce resources in Valemount and nearby communities like McBride. "There's not enough doctors in either community to sustain twenty-four seven coverage," Markham told me. "After hours, we [sometimes] cover McBride, and sometimes McBride will cover us." It was an early stage in the development of what Markham calls a "community of communities." I'll get to what that means and why he believes the concept is critical to the sustainability of healthcare in underserviced communities a bit later.

"I believe in virtual care," said Markham, who is the executive director of the Rural Coordination Centre of BC, or RCCbc, a network of hundreds of rural doctors and other healthcare providers and administrators, community members, policymakers, educators, researchers and non-profit and business leaders whose mission is to improve the health of people in rural communities. "But I'm going to say we've stubbed our toes many times in this whole process."

On one of those occasions, around twelve years ago, the RCCbc launched a partnership between a small local ER and the one in the larger hospital in Prince George. This pilot program was not unlike VERRa, in that a remote physician was communicating with staff at the smaller hospital using an iPad and Zoom. But unlike the VERRa docs, the ER physicians in Prince George were still on duty and had to juggle providing virtual consulting advice while taking care of in-person patients as well. "It was a dismal failure," Markham recalled.

But this early misstep led organizers to pivot from having ER physicians simultaneously working virtually and on-site to doing virtual shifts only, like the shifts Dr. Ertel does. That way, they are able to devote their full attention to their virtual duties. That was a game-changer. Now the rural doctors no longer have to wait in a long queue behind in-person patients in need of care. Instead, they get almost instant access to the virtual consultant. "We try and get online within twenty seconds of the button being pushed," said Markham.

Without in-person patients to treat, the virtual physician can also spend as much time as needed providing advice. Markham told me that in some instances, that has meant remaining on the virtual call for an hour or two, offering guidance on anything from how to stitch up a complicated laceration to how best to manage a patient who is having a cardiac arrest. Virtual physicians who aren't distracted by the need to respond to in-person emergencies are also less likely to see the request for advice as a burden and more likely to want to be helpful. "That is the fundamental difference," Markham told me.

Small ERs across the country are hanging by a thread. With dwindling numbers of family doctors, many of those ERs are but one sick nurse away from closing.

Whether they *should* stay open is another question entirely. Publicly, almost no one is prepared to argue that small ERs should close in favour of redirecting resources to larger regional hospitals. Few physicians want to say that any ER should shutter its doors. Instead, they and other healthcare leaders state ruefully that ERs should close if the provincial government is not prepared to make them more viable through increased spending.

Tim Vine, president and CEO of North Shore Health Network, told CBC News in December 2024, "We need help from policymakers and from planners within the system to determine whether or not there ought to be an emergency department in a particular location." North Shore manages three rural Ontario hospitals serving communities along northern Lake Huron. "I've got my answer, and it's an unequivocal yes," Vine added, "but if that's to be the case, we need to be funded in order to deliver that service."

In the same article, Al Drummond, who has advocated forcefully to make ERs both big and small sustainable, said, "Those days of every small town having an emergency department are regrettably over until we can develop some resilience in our health-care system."

Few politicians in Canada want to risk the political fallout that comes from closing small hospitals. They would much rather bask in the public adulation of reopening a previously closed ER. Recently, Manitoba Premier Wab Kinew made good on his promise to officials in the community of Carberry to reopen a small ER and hospital that were closed after the last family doctor left town. On the face of it, this seemed like a rare good news story about healthcare service in Canada. But privately, an official with the regional health authority that manages the newly reopened hospital told me it made more sense to close the ten-bed hospital and its four-stretcher ER permanently and convert the space to a long-term care home.

"Politically, nobody wants to go there, and I understand that," Dr. Mike Ertel told me. "But do we need all the emergency departments that we have now? No, we don't." Ertel isn't speaking only as a clinician. For more than five years, he was a vice president with Interior Health, a BC regional health authority. "At Interior Health, we did talk about closing some ERs in some of the smaller towns and would have been well within our rights to do so." But no one had the stomach to face the fallout. They saw the logic of closing some hospitals but did not want to deal with the political repercussions.

Lately, small ERs have been "closing themselves," Ertel said, due to acute shortages of nurses and physicians. But those closures are sporadic and temporary. Closing small-town hospitals permanently would have immediate and long-term consequences—and not just for healthcare. "If you lose your hospital, you probably lose your teachers and your bankers, and you can lose your talent," Ertel said. "You lose your young people because you can't have a baby there. You can't be confident that your child is going to get good medical care without the hospital."

Dr. Lindsey Dobson told me that she and her colleagues in Mackenzie have moulded their practices to the presence of a local hospital. Because there are no specialists in town, the seven family doctors who live and work there do "all things for all people." They work as ER physicians. They admit patients with pneumonia and other general internal medicine problems. They do procedures such as biopsies and draining fluid from the chest to see if the fluid contains cancer cells. "We couldn't do this type of practice if we didn't have the hospital facilities to back [us] up," she noted.

When I began writing this book, I assumed that closing small ERs was the fiscally sensible thing to do. It turns out that is not the only way of looking at things. There is an emerging counterargument that small ERs in rural and remote parts of Canada should be kept open, and maybe even expanded.

"I'll say absolutely that is the direction I think we should be going," Dr. Ray Markham told me. He believes that patients should receive their tests and treatments as close to home as possible. Closing smaller ERs means people must travel long distances to regional hospitals to get diagnostic testing and receive care.

"In British Columbia, we really struggle with transporting patients out of rural communities," Markham said. People have to be driven over mountains and on highways in all kinds of weather, with all of the attendant hazards. Markham startled me by saying that there is a calculable mortality rate for ordering, say, a CT scan in a hospital two to three hours away by car.

"I've had a patient and a family member die on their way to a routine scan," he told me. "We've had ambulances go off the road with patients in them."

Even when the transport goes off without a hitch, there are issues for the system. Towns like Mackenzie and Valemount rely on small cadres of physicians, nurses and paramedics to provide care. When a patient requires site-to-site transport, it means that at least one member of the team will be unavailable for hours and sometimes even a day or two. "The transport system is currently not nearly good enough to be able to move people at the drop of a hat," Markham said

Then there's the social cost to patients of being taken hours away from their homes to receive care. The long distances between the big hospital and their homes means friends and family are less likely to be present to support them. "Pulling people out of the community and their supportive networks and dropping them into big centres causes a lot of harm," said Markham.

Proponents of augmenting healthcare resources at small rural hospitals also argue that parts of rural BC contribute substantially to the province's GDP. They believe it's time healthcare catches up to that reality. "Rural areas are often the economic juggernaut for provinces," said Lindsey Dobson. "If you take away medical access in these places, you take away a good portion of the means of the province's GDP. I don't think the solution is closing down hospitals and medical resources in small towns."

Markham believes that virtual care will play a huge role in bringing higher levels of expertise to remote parts of the province. "In

British Columbia, we're moving into hybrid care," he told me. "I think it's super important that there is somebody physically in person in the community. [But] there are also times when that's not available . . . I think [virtual support] is a good thing, and I think people can get better care in those environments when they have both." Markham also believes that having a virtual option will make it easier to attract and retain younger physicians.

There is no question that some towns can go from sustainable to unsustainable with the departure of just one MD. This is why Markham is also a proponent of the "community of communities" approach mentioned earlier. He believes that small towns that border one another should band together to share resources, including physicians, as they've done in Valemount and McBride. He believes those kinds of collaborations should happen throughout the province. And in all provinces, for that matter.

"How do you create critical mass and economies of scale?" Markham asks. "Those things are going to be more and more important, particularly as we look at the economics and the costs of delivering healthcare in Canada. I think they are achievable in rural areas, but you do need to be working on that, actually and intentionally."

Ertel told me he likes the model Markham is describing but says there will be times when patients must be transported to hospitals with greater expertise and resources. "Our transport system is not as reliable as we would like it to be," he said. "If we have better transport and better virtual care, I think it can be done. I think it's the future."

The future that Ertel envisions includes physicians like Dr. Nic Sparrow, the orange-jumpsuited emergency medical services physician I met in BC. As Sparrow drives around the Kootenay region rescuing sick and injured people at the scene, he's effectively bringing the ER to patients. Sparrow is doing something that should be replicated in the farthest and most remote parts of Canada. And

Dr. Michael Christian may well be the one to make that happen. As I write this, he and several colleagues are working on a vastly scaled-up version of what Nic Sparrow is doing called Med Response BC.

Christian's plan involves a three-pronged approach. The first is to expand the type of service Sparrow provides by training and equipping MDs throughout the province. The second is to advance the development of search and rescue services in the province to model what's done in places like the United Kingdom. The third is to bring to Canada a new kind of medicine called retrieval medicine, which involves deploying a medical team, by land or air, to provide advanced and expert care of seriously ill and injured patients at the scene of an accident or at a healthcare facility like a remote nursing station or a small ER.

Retrieval medicine, as practised in Australia and Scotland, is all about caring for patients where they live. Christian told me that roughly a third of the patients that the Scottish retrieval team treats are able to remain in their communities. "The team will go there, they'll diagnose, they'll do the ultrasound, and they'll find out what they can do," he explained. "They'll support the local clinicians to provide care to that patient, stabilize them, and then, when appropriate, leave them there, often supported by telemedicine." It's a marriage of technology and skilled emergency personnel that reaches patients where they live, no matter how remote.

Dr. Mike Ertel sees an almost limitless future for technology and medicine. "Someday, virtual care will be people diagnosing themselves at home," he told me. "Whether it's taking their own blood or [operating] some scanner—we're just scratching the surface. In ten years, it's going to be something we don't even think about now. It's going to be people at home talking to their family doctor or cardiologist."

In other words, some patients won't need to come to the ER. The ER will come to them.

EPILOGUE

For now, we need and will continue to need ERs made of bricks and mortar. But as we've seen throughout the book, those in-person ERs, large and small, are seeing more patients than they can properly handle. The patients who visit those ERs fill every stretcher in every hallway. When they run out of stretchers, the patients fill every chair in the waiting room.

Some have called the current situation in emergency medicine a "collapse." That term may well describe your local ER if it is so overwhelmed that it can no longer cope with patients in need of immediate care. The term "crisis point" may more accurately describe ERs that are unable to see most patients in anything approaching a reasonable period of time, and those that are routinely required to care for patients in hallways and waiting rooms.

In Canada, we have certainly reached a moment of crisis, an inflection point in the viability and sustainability of emergency medicine as we know it.

The emergency departments that arose with acute care hospitals after the Second World War were built to stabilize and care for critically ill and injured patients. Over the years, their mandate has expanded to include the diagnosis of acute illnesses regardless of the immediate threat to life. As a critical part of society's safety net, the ER cares for the most vulnerable members of society, including people with severe mental health disease, alcohol and drug dependence and precarious housing. More recently, ERs have become the landing spot for the growing number of Canadians who lack primary care.

We have taken on those patients, sometimes with passion and sometimes as part of the job. But every system has its limits. In the years to come, we will test those limits with emerging infections like Covid and avian flu. Unfortunately, we are also seeing the re-emergence of older pathogens. In 1998, the World Health Organization declared that Canada had eliminated measles. In 2024 and 2025, Canada has seen significant outbreaks of measles in New Brunswick, Quebec, Ontario and Alberta. The latter two provinces have had case counts not seen in this country since the 1980s. By the middle of 2025, Canada had recorded more than four thousand cases of measles and climbing, three times more cases than the entire US.

The reasons are severalfold. Dramatically lower rates of immunization with the measles, mumps and rubella (MMR) vaccine abroad mean huge outbreaks in other countries. An increased number of visitors from countries that have active outbreaks are arriving in Canada in the early stages of measles, before the typical rash appears. Declining rates of MMR immunization in this country due to vaccine skepticism mean that infected visitors stand a greater chance of infecting people living here, leading to local outbreaks.

In Canada, as many as 27 per cent of people infected with measles have required hospitalization. Their increasing need for hospitals guarantees greater demand for the ER.

And it's not just new and old infections that will bring many more patients to Canada's emergency departments. So too will environmental disasters caused by climate change. On June 6, 2025, Toronto briefly recorded the worst air quality in the world. The cause was wildfire smoke that had spread across the province. At the time, fifteen out-of-control wildfires had been burning in northern Ontario and western Canada. The wildfire smoke prompted Environment Canada to issue a special air quality statement for the GTA and much of southern Ontario, as well as five other provinces.

The symptoms of wildfire smoke exposure include coughing, shortness of breath, wheezing, chest pains, difficulty breathing, burning eyes, runny nose, dizziness, headaches, heart palpitations and fatigue. The smoke worsens pre-existing conditions such as asthma, chronic obstructive pulmonary disease, heart disease and heart failure. Pregnant women are more likely to have miscarriages or give birth to infants with low birth weight. People with weakened immune systems are more vulnerable to complications from smoke exposure.

With no end in sight, wildfire smoke is bound to cause huge spikes in ER visits. As is, emergency departments have no slack. The system is asking the people who work there to do too much. ER physicians, nurses and other providers have complained bitterly about this. But few if any have taken concrete steps to push back. Dr. Kaitlin Stockton is a notable exception. That's because she took the unprecedented step of suing the health authority that runs the two hospitals where she worked for more than seven years.

Stockton, who is thirty-nine years old, graduated from the University of Toronto Faculty of Medicine before doing postgraduate residency training in Family Medicine and Emergency Medicine at UBC. She lives in North Vancouver with her husband (an orthopedic surgeon) and their two kids. From October 2017 until recently, Stockton was an ER physician at Royal Columbian Hospital (RCH) in New Westminster and Eagle Ridge Hospital (ERH) in Port Moody. Both BC hospitals are run by Fraser Health Authority (FHA).

On June 6, 2025, Stockton filed a Notice of Civil Claim (Claim) with the B.C. Supreme Court against FHA, alleging problems at both ERH and RCH. The lawsuit alleged that the FHA had ignored warnings from doctors and other staff about personnel and other shortages that led to unsafe conditions for patients and for the people who look after them.

According to the Claim, "Over the past two years, Dr. Stockton and her colleagues repeatedly advocated for FHA to respond to the deteriorating working conditions at both Hospitals and to increasingly unsafe and substandard patient care due to overcapacity and resource shortage issues." Stockton alleged that the working conditions at both hospitals were "physically, psychologically, and clinically unsafe, leading to severe and preventable harm to patients, physicians, and other medical staff." The Claim also alleged that "FHA has ignored these efforts and done little to nothing to improve working conditions."

The Claim cited seven episodes in which Stockton alleged that ER nurses or physicians were attacked verbally or physically by patients, including one episode in which an ER staff physician claimed to have been attacked "by a patient's large Pitbull that was allegedly allowed to enter the ER at ERH and remain in an open area with other patients for several hours."

The Claim alleged that "despite repeated efforts of many ER doctors at FHA, working conditions in the Hospitals' ERs have continued to deteriorate."

None of these claims were tested in court. FHA did not file a statement of defence, but instead in July 2025, they filed a Jurisdictional Response to the lawsuit, disputing that the court had jurisdiction and that it "ought not to exercise its jurisdiction over the defendant."

"Fraser Health doesn't comment on matters that are before the courts," Krystle Landert, a senior consultant in public affairs with FHA, told me. In an article published June 25, 2025 (following the initial coverage of Stockton's lawsuit), the authority provided a statement in response to inquiries from CBC News regarding violent incidents that were cited in Stockton's Claim. "We are deeply concerned about the violent incidents that occurred at Eagle Ridge Hospital in November 2024 and January 2025 and the impact it had on staff and medical staff," the authority wrote. "In March 2025, we increased security staffing in the Emergency Department at Eagle Ridge Hospital in direct response to recent violent incidents. We also strengthened training for site security and increased on-the-floor coaching to ensure staff are fully prepared to respond effectively."

As this book was going to print, Stockton announced on X that her legal matter with FHA had been resolved. She did not share the terms of the resolution except to say that she was "satisfied with the outcome." FHA confirmed that the matter had been resolved to the parties' mutual satisfaction, again without further details.

Stockton's statement on X went on to say that she had pursued the case "guided by the conviction that healthcare workers deserve a safe and respectful workplace where we can fulfill our essential roles as medical experts, caregivers, leaders, and advocates. Advocating for patients, ourselves, and the integrity of our healthcare system is our professional and ethical obligation, and we must remain free to do so without fear of censorship or retaliation."

In its own statement FHA said it "appreciates the role our staff and medical staff play in providing safe, high-quality and compassionate care to our patients and communities, and remain committed to making our workplaces as safe as possible for all staff, medical staff, patients and families." In expressing its commitment to improve key workplace policies especially relating to a safe and respectful workplace, FHA said it "remains committed to fostering a culture where staff and medical staff who identify safety concerns or advocate for system improvements are heard, supported, and engaged in a collaborative manner."

Stockton's case was actually framed as a claim for constructive dismissal so we do not know if any part of the settlement concerned patient safety or working conditions. Still, I think it's important to include this story in the book because it was arguably the first time an emergency physician in Canada sued a health authority in a way that sought to put the issue of patient and provider safety under the litigation spotlight.

What compelled Stockton to take that momentous step? In an interview when she filed the claim, Stockton said she saw three potential courses of action in response to the issues she and colleagues dealt with at the two FHA hospitals where she worked. "You can put this behind you and move on with your life," she told me. "You can work the internal channels and get more involved in leadership and internal advocacy. Or, you can sue them and do something that maybe has never been done before, is risky, but has the potential of setting legal precedent and making a permanent, positive change for the profession, the patients and the country."

Stockton received institutional support from emergency colleagues. "Without commenting on the merits of her litigation specifically, we support Dr. Stockton's right to pursue her case through legal avenues if necessary," wrote Drs. Jonathan Braunstein, Garth Meckler and Ben Tuyp, copresidents of the BC Society of Emergency Medicine. The BCSEM represents over 750 emergency physicians in the province. The Alberta Medical Association's Section of Emergency Medicine, which represents over 600 emergency physicians working in communities and hospitals across Alberta, said, "We are writing to express our solidarity with Dr. Kaitlin Stockton, an emergency physician in British Columbia, and to raise awareness about the silencing and intimidation of physicians who advocate for patient safety and system reform."

As well, the Saskatchewan Medical Association Section of

Emergency Medicine wrote a statement to express its solidarity with Stockton, "and to draw urgent attention to the concerning pattern of silencing and intimidation faced by physicians who advocate for patient safety and system reform."

Stockton's kind of courage will be necessary if we are to make the changes that will be necessary to put emergency medicine on a surer footing.

ERs will continue to be necessary to stabilize and treat patients with life-threatening illnesses and injuries, although we will undoubtedly treat more of those emergencies in the field or at the scene. For the patients who come to the ER because they have no other more appropriate place to go, the solution is to create those better places.

A 2024 report by the Canadian Institute for Health Information found that between April 2023 and March 2024, one in seven visits to ERs in Canada were for conditions that could potentially have been managed by a family doctor or a nurse practitioner.

It seems obvious to assume that unattached patients will use the ER far less if they have a family doctor or nurse practitioner to consult. To that end, new medical schools are opening up in several provinces. One of the most intriguing is Queen's-Lakeridge Health MD Family Medicine Program, Canada's first medical school training program for family doctors only. It's a creative initiative, but with just twenty students per year, it will take a long time for a school like this to fill the gap in any meaningful way.

There have been calls to fast-track doctors (including ER physicians) from other countries, especially the US. In the months since the second Trump administration, a growing number of American physicians have either moved to Canada or have expressed a keen interest in doing so. Ontario has taken steps to make it easier for doctors and nurses licensed in the US to work for up to six months while applying for a provincial licence (and their landed immigrant status). BC is working with its provincial college to license doctors who are certified in the US without requiring them to complete further assessments, training or examination. Nova Scotia and New Brunswick are among the provinces following a similar path.

This is a one-time opportunity to benefit from physician unrest in the US. However, like all gold mines, this one will soon become exhausted.

The Canadian Medical Association and other organizations have called for a pan-Canadian licence for healthcare professionals. That would facilitate the movement of ER physicians and other ER providers across Canada. In theory, a pan-Canadian license would allow the movement of ER providers from provinces that are well stocked to those in need. It could also have the opposite effect by causing the movement of providers to provinces that have the resources to pay them higher fees.

In the meantime, there are other things provinces can do to boost primary care in the short term, including fast-tracking the credentialing of doctors from other countries and training nurse practitioners to practise primary care independently, as has been done with success in Ontario since 2008. This will increase the supply of primary care providers, but even then, there is no guarantee that every Canadian who wants a family doctor will get one, and no guarantee that those who have one will get quick and easy access to appointments. To address those issues, Canada should borrow ideas from other countries with a better track record.

In January 2025, I travelled to Denmark, where more than 98 per cent of people have family doctors. Both Denmark and Canada have publicly funded healthcare systems, but Denmark also permits doctors to go private.

The first thing I learned is that Denmark prioritizes primary care in several ways. For one thing, general practitioners, or GPs, get paid more than family doctors in Canada. But it's more than a matter of money. In Denmark, GPs play a critical role as the gatekeepers of the healthcare system. You don't get an appointment with a specialist unless you go through a GP. And while you can go to the nearest ER, you won't be seen unless you have a life- or limb-threatening injury or illness. Instead, you'll be directed to call your own GP or the emergency medical service for further advice.

But the most important way Denmark shows that it values primary care is by providing a GP to each person who is eligible through a mandatory enrollment program. If you think that sounds odd or impossible to engineer, remember that in Canada's public education system, your kids are automatically enrolled in a school based on where you live. In Denmark, both your kids' school and your GP are determined by your address. In fact, the name of your GP is printed right at the top of your Central Person Register card, which is similar to a Canadian social insurance number card.

Another thing I noticed in Denmark is how well they do teamwork in primary care. I visited a clinic in Frederiksberg, an independent municipality in the heart of Copenhagen. There, I saw GPs, nurses and midwives working seamlessly with an efficient division of labour. GPs see patients with acute as well as complex medical problems. Nurses see patients with chronic ailments like diabetes and hypertension. Midwives provide prenatal care and see women with gynecological problems, as well as kids. These professionals work contentedly alongside one another. They don't compete for patients.

And Denmark is not the only EU country that does something well worth emulating. The Netherlands has an outstanding system of urgent after-hours primary care delivered by phone or video. The service is available between 5:00 p.m. and 8:00 a.m. on weekdays, as well as on weekends and holidays. The program is run by GPs called *huisartsenposten*, or house doctors.

How it works is that a patient will call their GP's office as usual. In the message they hear, there's an option to request urgent medical care. The urgent care call centre is staffed by two GPs who supervise several practice assistants. These are healthcare providers with medical training whose role is to triage the calls using algorithms. If the issue is life-threatening, the practice assistant sends an ambulance. Patients who do not have emergencies but need to be seen in person are sent to an after-hours clinic close to where they live. The supervising GPs sign off on every call.

Like Denmark, the Netherlands doesn't allow you to just show up at an ER and expect to be treated unless you have a life-threatening emergency. In both countries, the default is that your GP or someone providing urgent after-hours care is responsible for your well-being twenty-four hours a day, seven days a week.

To make that system work in Canada, we would need both mandatory enrollment in primary care and universal after-hours access. We would also need to forbid patients from selecting the ER for care when an illness or injury is not immediately life-threatening. These things require a seismic shift in what we do now. Over the years, I have seen lots of patients who get misdiagnosed on the first visit to the ER and get the correct diagnosis and treatment on a subsequent visit. That said, I have also seen many patients return to the ER multiple times for assessment and treatment of the same medical complaint, receiving the same diagnosis at each visit. We have all seen lots of patients who get discharged from one hospital only to visit another in search of a new diagnostic workup and a different result.

Doctors in Denmark might find this laissez-faire system of ER access we have in Canada expensive and unhelpful to patients. I believe it has reached the point of unsustainability. Other countries restrict ER access and don't seem to have worse outcomes. This isn't outside-the-box thinking. It's trying something different that works elsewhere.

That said, I have serious doubts that Canada will follow the lead of countries like Denmark and the Netherlands anytime soon. For one thing, it would require a tax increase, and that by itself would likely be a deal-breaker. Another issue is that the provinces have jurisdiction over healthcare. Some provinces are trying to link each of their residents with a primary care provider. For instance, in January 2025, the Ontario government announced an investment of $1.8 billion to connect two million Ontario residents to a publicly funded family doctor or primary care team within four years. That effort, dubbed Ontario's Primary Care Action Team, is led by Dr. Jane Philpott, a renowned family doctor, former federal minister of health, and former dean of the Faculty of Health Sciences and director of the School of Medicine at Queen's University in Kingston, Ontario.

Still, it's hard to imagine every province agreeing to guarantee all of its residents timely access to family medicine. We might be more likely to see the emergence of private for-profit healthcare than the reforms I'm talking about. In Quebec, already a small but growing number of primary care doctors have opted out of the public system to provide private family medicine. I met one doctor who charges patients $150 for a fifteen-minute appointment, $300 for a thirty-minute appointment, and so on. He generally offers same- or next-day appointments, which is almost unheard of in the public system. In response, the province has proposed legislation to force new doctors to practise in the public system for five years after they graduate, and to make it harder for physicians already in practice to go private.

To improve healthcare access across the board, we need to develop better places for unhoused people and those with substance use disorders and chronic mental health disease to seek treatment. Forward-thinking healthcare systems in Canada are finally beginning to organize alternatives to the ER. As we saw earlier in the book, University Health Network in Toronto has a pilot program to provide stable housing and comprehensive social and health services to patients identified as frequent visitors to the ER. There is no reason why other cities and even entire provinces can't provide similar supports for vulnerable Canadians. The key, in my opinion, is for authorities to stop thinking of the ER as the great undifferentiated place where everybody goes when they can't find help anywhere else. When people have a better alternative than going to the ER, it's a win for the ER and a win for the patients.

Measures like these will reduce the strain on Canada's ERs by decreasing the number of patients coming to the hospital. The other way to reduce wait times and address hallway medicine is to help patients move through the ER more quickly. Dr. Al Drummond has said repeatedly over decades that more beds in long-term care facilities frees up beds on hospital wards, which in turn allows ER patients to be transferred to the wards sooner so they no longer have to spend days languishing in hallways.

Better and more comprehensive home care services would also mean that more patients can be safely discharged instead of being admitted to the hospital. All provinces should expand services to allow stable patients to receive more advanced care in their own homes. In the United Kingdom, it's not unusual for multidisciplinary teams to provide intensive, hospital-level care at home for conditions that would normally require an acute care hospital bed.

This is a time for bold ideas, and many of the boldest ideas for reimagining emergency medicine are coming from ER physicians themselves. For all the talk of burnout, these colleagues maintain a passion for ER medicine that simply refuses to die. It's also noteworthy how many of those innovative notions are coming from the growing number of women working in ERs across Canada. Dr. Keerat Grewal is helping to define the growing trend to diagnose cancer in the ER and is working on ways to help those patients get the biopsies and other tests they need so they can receive the most appropriate care. Dr. Catherine Varner is developing a model that provides aftercare and emotional support for the one in five women whose pregnancy ends in a miscarriage.

To all of this, let me add one more important prescription. The new generation of ER physicians is brilliant, dedicated, resourceful and kind. They are the people you want running the place inside the sliding doors. It is well past time for ER physicians in hospitals big and small to be in charge of their own house. It means that they should be the primary setters of policy on patient capacity and safety in the emergency department. Until now, the people who work in ERs have largely been forced to increase capacity almost limitlessly in response to shocks elsewhere in the system. And we've done this as if there are no limits to our capacity to see patients in a timely fashion when there are frequent and glaring examples to the contrary.

Dr. Kaitlin Stockton is a member of that younger vanguard who believe enough is enough. "As a specialty, we need to set some standards," she told me. "We need to set some boundaries where we say, 'No, this is unacceptable.'"

And unlike other ER physicians, Stockton has thought about where to draw the line. "Emergency departments should have the golden rule whereby seventy-five per cent of our beds are reserved for ER patients," she told me when we talked in the summer of 2025. "Twenty-five per cent of the beds can be for admitted patients."

And she has other ideas. "We need to have a certain number of nurses to operate safely," she adds. "We need to have a standard of care to which we are held accountable and which is actually enforced. We also need to be treated respectfully. We need to feel safe. We need to not be harassed."

From my earliest days as an ER doctor more than four decades ago, we have revelled in our ability to 'MacGyver' our way to saving patients. Stockton thinks we've taken that capacity to its limits.

"We're great at filling the cracks with grout and keeping the boat afloat," she says. "Because we've been so great at being innovative and adaptable, we've kept the boat afloat this long. Except now the boat is just so full of people that the whole thing's going to sink."

I hope Stockton and others like her become the new leaders of emergency medicine. I look forward to the day when hospital executives and colleagues on the wards, in the OR and in the ICU as well as hospital leaders defer to ER personnel on matters that pertain to patient flow within the ER itself. For they are the ones who know best how to keep the light on in the lighthouse.

7:05 a.m.

The back entrance to the hospital bustles with the arrival of the day shift. The day people are rested, fed and caffeinated to start the morning. They have an energy that I can't match right now. I nod to the security guards as I go through the revolving door to exit the hospital.

The initial blast of winter air as I leave the building is bracing. To the east, the first rays of orange sunlight sneak between tall buildings. A wailing siren grows louder. For a moment, I stop walking in case the ambulance is coming to my ER. I think about returning to help out but quickly remember that my colleagues can handle things.

The receding sound of the siren reminds me that my time in the ER grows short. Although I complain about the hours and the stress, I will miss being at the centre of the action. I'm already envious of Samir, Tawny, Fix and all my younger colleagues, whose most productive years lie ahead. Ahu most of all because she is just getting started.

As I enter the concrete stairwell of the covered parking lot across from the hospital, all I can think of is driving home while I'm awake enough to navigate the perpetual traffic jams on the streets of Toronto.

I climb the steps and soon can hear a faint hubbub coming from a couple of flights above me. It's indistinct at first, but with each step I climb, it becomes more rhythmic and more familiar.

"Fifteen, sixteen, seventeen, eighteen, nineteen, twenty . . ."

I quicken my pace as the sound gets clearer and more distinct.

"Help! Help!" a voice issues forth from the top of the stairs.

"Ahu, is that you?" I call out, breathless as I climb two steps at a time until I reach the top.

Ahu is bent over a man doing CPR. I can't see the man's face, but I can make out the sleeve of a sequined rainbow-coloured tuxedo jacket. Joseph left the ER in a hurry but didn't get far.

"What have you got?" I slip back into attending physician mode, joining her in a two-person basic life support rescue.

"He was down when I found him," she says. "Non-responsive, no pulse, no respirations, pinpoint pupils. I called 911 ten minutes ago. Still waiting for the crew."

"Here, maybe this will help." I pull a naloxone kit from my coat pocket.

Ahu looks incredulous. "You carry it?"

"I didn't always." I open the package and take out a syringe and an alcohol pad. "A colleague says he never leaves home without it. He figures he's saved half a dozen people in the past two years."

"Do you mind?" Ahu stops me as I'm about to inject the opioid antidote into the deltoid muscle in Joseph's left shoulder.

"He's your patient," I tell her as I take over chest compressions.

Ahu injects the syringe's contents in one brisk motion, then places a couple of fingers on the right side of Joseph's neck so she can feel the carotid artery for a pulse. "Come on, Theo. Wake up."

My post–casino shift sleepiness is gone. I pour myself into pressing rhythmically onto Joseph's chest. "Come on," I whisper.

In the distance, I catch the faint sound of a siren.

"Listen," I tell Ahu as the sound gets closer and my chest compressions grow stronger. Suddenly, the siren stops, and we hear what sounds like the back door of an ambulance slamming shut.

"Hello, can you hear me?" a female voice calls out. "Where are you?'

"We're in the stairwell four flights up from street level," I yell out.

"We're on our way up," says the voice.

"I've got a pulse!" Ahu says loudly. "Stop compressions but continue rescue breathing."

"Well, I might have known I'd see you two here," Virginia huffs as she reaches the top of the stairs bearing a case of equipment. Her partner, Tom, is following close behind.

Virginia takes out a blood pressure cuff and wraps it around Joseph's arm. Tom puts ECG leads on Joseph's chest and an oxygen saturation clip on his thumb. He presses the power button on the portable heart monitor he and Virginia hauled upstairs.

"Heart rate 116 and regular," says Tom. "BP 105 over 70. Resps are 9 and O_2 sat is 92."

"Nice save, Doctor," says Virginia.

"That was Ahu," I quickly correct her.

"We had the dream team," says Ahu. "Hey, Theo, wake up!" She presses a knuckle on his chest until his eyes open.

"Does he need another dose of naloxone?" I ask her.

"Let's not make his dope sickness any worse," she replies.

"We'll watch him carefully for signs of unresponsiveness," says Virginia. She and Tom lift Joseph onto a portable stretcher they brought upstairs.

"If you don't mind, I'd like to bring him back to the ER," says Ahu. "He's my patient. Brian, you look tired. You should go home and get some sleep."

I watch Ahu, Virginia and Tom roll the stretcher bearing Joseph into the parking lot elevator. As the doors close, Ahu shoots me a quick glance. She's got tears in her eyes. I've been where she is. Sleep deprivation is a bit like alcohol; it uncorks your emotions. Maybe it's tears of triumph. Maybe it's tears of relief that Joseph won't die on her watch. At least not this time.

For a moment, I want to follow them to the ER. But that will be Ahu's story to tell, not mine.

ACKNOWLEDGEMENTS

My name may be the only one on the cover of *The Casino Shift*, but there is no conceivable way I could have written it without a lot of help.

Fellow journalists Karin Chykaliuk and Emily Mathieu helped me plot the general direction and broad content of the book. Karin sourced some of my most vivid interviews in my previous book, *The Power of Kindness,* and I was grateful that she came back to help fulfill the same role in *The Casino Shift*. Whenever my energy flagged, she was there to remind me that the stories in this book are worth knowing and the book's message is timely. Emily also found several essential sources for the book. She has a knack for distilling large government reports into their elemental bits. She did so on the *Public Inquiry Commission on Relations between Indigenous Peoples and Certain Public Services in Québec* (the Viens Commission) and sourced the testimony of Natasia Mukash, mother of Jade Mukash.

I want to thank my editor at HarperCollins, Brad Wilson, for asking me to write a sequel to *The Night Shift*. His unwavering enthusiasm sustained me through the months of researching and writing the book. When I told Brad that I needed to make the tone of the book more serious than that of *The Night Shift* to reflect the moment, his support was unconditional.

Janice Weaver and Nicole Langlois both helped wrestle the book down to a more manageable length and into the readable form in which you have found it. Thanks to Shaun Oakey for his detailed copyedit. I want to thank Jim Gifford, my original editor on *The Night Shift*, for helping me develop the voice that made its debut in that book and that I have carried into this one.

Once again, my colleagues Colleen Ross, Jennifer Warren, Stephanie Dubois and Sameer Chhabra at *White Coat, Black Art* and *The Dose* provided a sounding board for my thoughts on the book and a lot of encouragement. I am grateful to Stephanie for introducing me to Drs. Nic Sparrow, Mike Ertel and Lindsey Dobson. Their interviews formed the backbone of the sections on KERPA and virtual emergency medicine. I also want to thank Jennifer for introducing me to Muskoka paramedic Stuart McKinnon, who provided essential comments on the opioid crisis in Ontario's cottage country.

I could not begin to tell the story of emergency medicine in Canada without the support of my colleagues across Canada. Their names are too numerous to mention here, but I want to single out Lorri Beatty, Ian Chernoff, Lindsey Dobson, Mike Ertel, Keerat Grewal, Trevor Jain, Ken Milne, Carolyn Snider, Qassim Tejpar, Catherine Varner and Raghu Venugopal for their generous and eye-opening contributions to this book.

I am grateful to Dr. Alan Drummond for inviting me to Perth to see how it's possible to deliver first-order care in a tiny rural hospital.

Words cannot fully express my admiration for the doctors, nurses, respiratory therapists, social workers, pharmacists, physical and occupational therapists, residents and students with whom I have had the privilege of working during the past four decades. They are the true heroes of the ER.

As always, I am grateful to my agent Rick Broadhead, who has nurtured my career as a book author.

To my kids, Kaille and Alex, who love to hear their dad spin tales from the ER, and who wait ever patiently for him to emerge from his writing sessions in the basement office.

To my wife, Tamara, who knows all of my secrets and who, thanks to our nightly neighbourhood walks, knows everything I'm going to write before I write it.

June 8, 2025